The Pancreatic Oath

The Pancreatic Oath

Based on the Pancreatic Nutritional Program™

*The measurable approach
to improved health and weight loss*

*A Common Sense Approach
to Sustained Health*

Candice P. Rosen, R.N., B.S., M.S.W., C.H.C.

NOTICE: This publication is intended to provide helpful information and dietary tips, advice and suggestions, intended only to assist readers with interest in obtaining information regarding dietary changes. It is not intended to diagnose, treat, cure or prevent any health condition or concern. Neither the publisher nor the author is engaged in rendering professional medical advice or nutrition counseling services to the individual reader. The information provided in this book should not be interpreted as a substitute for a physician consultation, evaluation or treatment. Nothing written in this book should be construed as medical advice or diagnosis.

Before beginning any diet and/or exercise program, always consult with your physician or primary health care provider to ensure your health and safety. Any suggestions or inferences drawn from this book should be reviewed with a licensed medical professional before your implementation. The author and publisher will not be held responsible for individuals who intend and carry out harm to themselves or other individuals. The author, publisher, its agents and representatives shall not be held responsible for any information interpreted as such by any readers. The author, publisher, its agents and representatives specifically disclaim all responsibility for any liability, loss of risk, personal or otherwise, which may be incurred as a consequence, directly or indirectly, from the use or application of any contents of this book. The statements made in this book have not been evaluated by the Food and Drug Administration of the United States of America.

While all reasonable efforts have been made to ensure that all the information presented is accurate, as research and development in the nutrition and medical fields are ongoing, it is possible that new findings may supersede some of the data presented. While the author has made every effort to provide accurate web addresses at the time of publication, neither the publisher nor the author assumes any responsibility for errors, or for changes that occur after publication.

Mention of specific companies, organizations, or authorities in this book does not imply endorsement by the author or publisher, nor does mention of specific companies, organizations, or authorities imply their endorsement of this book, its author, or the publisher.

For information about this title or to order other books and/or electronic media, contact the publisher:

Pancreatic Nutritional Program, a division of Candice Rosen Health Counseling, LLC

info@pnprogram.com

www.pnprogram.com

Library of Congress Cataloguing-in-Publication Data

Rosen, Candice P.

Pancreatic Oath, The: measurable approach to improved health and weight loss/Candice P. Rosen

ISBN: 978-0-9836413-6-0 Hardcover

Printed in the United States of America

Cover and interior design: 1106 Design

This book is dedicated to

Melissa,
Jennifer,
Natalie, and
Nicholas.

My reasons for being.

Health Disclaimer

This publication is intended to provide helpful information and dietary tips, advice and suggestions, intended only to assist readers with interest in obtaining information regarding dietary changes. It is not intended to diagnose, treat, cure or prevent any health condition or concern. The information provided in this book should not be interpreted as a substitute for physician consultation, evaluation or treatment. Nothing written in this book should be construed as medical advice or diagnosis. Before beginning any diet and/or exercise program, always consult with your physician or primary health care provider to ensure your health and safety. Any suggestions or inferences drawn from this book should be reviewed with a licensed medical professional before your implementation. The author and publisher will not be held responsible for individuals who intend and carry out harm to themselves or other individuals.

The author, publisher, its agents and representatives shall not be held responsible for any information interpreted as such by any readers. The author, publisher, its agents and representatives specifically disclaim all responsibility for any liability, loss of risk, personal or otherwise, which may be incurred as a consequence, directly or indirectly, from the use or application of any contents of this book. The statements made in this book have not been evaluated by the Food and Drug Administration of the United States of America.

Table of Contents

A Letter to the Reader

Dear Reader,

The *Pancreatic Oath* is NOT a diet book. It is NOT a nutrition book. It is NOT a book for diabetics. It is NOT a self-help book. *The Pancreatic Oath* is a revolutionary *Self-Health* book. Yes, a ***Self-Health*** Book! After reading *The Pancreatic Oath*, you will be empowered with the knowledge of how to read the language of your body in order to best achieve your personal health and weight loss goals.

There is no "one size fits all" way of eating that reduces weight or prevents illness. That is probably why so many of us fail at dieting. We are all different and our bodies react differently to the food we ingest. Learning how *your* body reacts to food will give you the power to control your weight and your health. How do you learn the way in which your body will react to food? By listening to the lessons and the "language" spoken by your body.

Over the past seven years, I have taught people how to listen to their bodies and watched as that wisdom nourished and healed them. I developed the Pancreatic Nutritional Program™ (PNP) in response to my family's and my own health concerns. As I wrote *The Pancreatic Oath*, based on my program's success with clients, I began to see the great implications that the PNP had for the health care crisis in America and the growing global obesity epidemic. I truly believe my simple, yet innovative approach has remarkable implications for the fields of prevention medicine and nutritional healing.

There is nothing more precious than good health. Poor health is expensive. Even one chronic health condition can deplete a person's financial resources and diminish their quality of life. While we all know that nothing is more precious than good health, few of us seem to be able to attain or maintain good health. When poor health is caused by a catastrophic event, it is simply tragic. When poor health is the result of apathy, laziness, or poor food choices, it is sinful. Fortunately, when poor health is due to a lack of knowledge, it can be changed.

The majority of illnesses that plague people in Western societies stem from a lack of knowledge about body chemistry and the effect foods and beverages have on overall health and weight. Most people simply do not know how their bodies work. A lack of knowledge stands in the way of health and a healthy lifestyle. For people that do know a thing or two about their bodies, they often do not know how to apply that knowledge. Sure, not every disease can be controlled by what we eat; however, you might just be surprised at how many diseases are impacted by diet and lifestyle. For diseases that can be controlled, control lies in knowledge. First, we must be educated and then we must act. It is true—we are what we eat.

Having an abundant supply of reasonably priced food in developed countries is both a profound blessing and a hidden curse. The curse of easy, plentiful food is that eating has become too easy. Our bodies are designed to hold on to every calorie because for much of human history it was incredibly hard to find a constant supply of food. While there is certainly starvation and malnutrition in the world, starvation is not killing most Westerners. Overeating and eating the wrong foods is killing us. These behaviors cause weight gain and chronic illness by increasing blood glucose and overworking the pancreas. Virtually all of us struggle to reach or maintain our ideal body weight and preserve good health. It seems paradoxical, does it not? We have a limitless selection of foods, but tend to choose the wrong things. In truth, the alternatives are overwhelming and make menu planning a formidable task. While we recognize the importance of proper nutrition, the challenge is to determine what foods work for *you* and *your* health.

Over time, the struggle becomes a battle. The battle to improve and maintain your health, decrease chronic illness, increase quality of life, and extend life expectancy is waged each time you eat. The obstacles you will face include a stressed and hectic lifestyle, processed foods, refined carbohydrates, hydrogenated oil, trans fats, high fructose corn syrup, sugars (artificial and regular), and foods high in salt. This book does not put an end to this battle, but it arms you with the intelligence and weapons needed to win the battle every day. The knowledge you will gain from this book will arm you with an understanding of your body chemistry. Through continued proper nutrition based on the PNP style of eating, you will win the war.

The Pancreatic Oath evolved from my own personal experience and a sincere desire to help family and friends with a myriad of problems related to poor eating habits and pancreatic abuse. The insights gained from *The Pancreatic Oath* will enable you to lose weight, to be sure; and if that is your only goal, then you will reach it. But as I mentioned, this is not a diet book. It is a *Self-Health* book. *The Pancreatic Oath* contains the knowledge that I have used to prevent and reverse many chronic illnesses. Weight loss is almost a side-benefit! This book gives *you* greater control over your life and health. When the knowledge contained in this book is applied to your life, the costs of treating a chronic illness—measured in time, hassle, and money—will dramatically decrease. At the same time, because you will enjoy good health, your quality of life will increase just as dramatically.

The Pancreatic Oath peels away the mystery that surrounds the functioning of the often overlooked, but terribly important gland called the pancreas. The pancreas has a number of biological functions that play a central role in the struggle—the battle—with weight and poor health. *The Pancreatic Oath* explains the crucial function that a healthy and unabused pancreas provides in the long-term health of each and every one of us. Understanding the pancreas is not just a high school biology topic (even though this is where most of us receive a brief overview about the pancreas). Protecting your pancreas is so crucial to human health that I wish my book could be required reading for every adult, teenager, and child. As you will learn, pancreatic abuse leads to polycystic ovarian syndrome, insulin resistance, metabolic syndrome, pre-diabetes, and the universally feared chronic illness, diabetes mellitus. Pancreatic abuse also leads to obesity. Obesity is emerging and expanding (quite literally) as the chief risk factor in heart disease, stroke, and cancer.

The Pancreatic Oath provides an elementary, but comprehensive explanation of the function of the pancreas. Moreover, it explains how healthy food choices can protect the pancreas and promote health, whereas unhealthy food choices actually abuse the pancreas and destroy health.

During my career as a registered nurse, as a social worker, and as a health counselor now, I have come to understand the extent of the problem and the difficulty that countless people face in maintaining a regimen that works for them. As a result, I developed the Pancreatic Nutritional Program™ (PNP). I have experienced the benefits of the PNP first-hand by healing myself and teaching family members and clients how to improve their health and achieve weight loss results.

I am proud and humble to say the PNP approach is uniformly successful. Based on these results, each individual will learn to listen to the voice of their body/pancreas and understand what foods raise their blood glucose and place their pancreas in a stressful situation versus foods that promote healthy blood glucose levels and place the pancreas in "idle mode." Food selection will also have an effect on how much insulin your pancreas needs to produce to keep your body functioning. All of this might be confusing right now, but by the end of this book, you will be an expert on your own body and your own health. You will understand how to achieve the daily PNP goal— eating to keep your blood glucose level between 70 and 100.

Your goal is to protect your pancreas, and that goal can only be accomplished through eating the correct foods for your body. Improved health should be the byproduct of your new path. Please let me know how it works for you. I value your feedback (e-mail me at info@pnprogram.com). The PNP has worked for family, friends, clients, and me. I want it to work for you. If you would like to schedule a counseling session or begin a program with our practice, please visit www.PNPROGRAM.com for more information.

Live and eat not just for today. Eat for all the tomorrows! I wish you a long life of valued *Self-Health*.

A Letter to Healthcare Professionals

Dear Doctors, Nurses, and Other Overworked Healthcare Professionals,

Nutrition education was and continues to be limited for those enrolled in medical or nursing schools. A study, published in the April 2006 issue of the *American Journal of Clinical Nutrition*, concludes that "the amount of nutrition education in medical schools remains inadequate" even 20 years after a report from the National Academy of Sciences found that nutrition education programs in medical schools were "largely inadequate to meet the present and future demands of the medical profession."

In today's world of managed healthcare, time is limited. Our time seems to be completely consumed by efforts to heal, cure, and ease suffering. There is no arguing that one must keep up with the latest advances in healthcare. I implore you to consider advances in nutrition as one of those critical pursuits of knowledge.

I don't know about you, but I hated studying nutrition in nursing school. It was brief, but as far as I was concerned it was way too long. I remember how I would cringe when I heard the word "legume" uttered! I have come a long way since then. Circumstance forced me back to nutrition, to legumes, and learning the healing properties of a host of additional wholesome, responsibly grown foods.

Most healthcare professionals do advise their patients to "lose weight and exercise." However, most healthcare professionals are ill equipped to offer truly effective food, nutrition, and diet tips. So, the patient walks out of the office without a clear understanding of where to start. No precise prescription for diet and exercise is given. Although many patients leave with a number for the hospital dietician or nutritionist, they find that the dietician or nutritionist is in need of help, too. Too often, registered dieticians emphasize antiquated nutrition protocols rooted in calorie counting and an agenda advocated by the American Dietetic Association. With so many diets, diet books, diet experts, where does one begin? Well, they usually don't. Frustrated, they stop off for a lunch or dinner of fast food after their appointment.

We know many health conditions, such as cancer, diabetes, and kidney disease, are related to what we eat. *The Pancreatic Oath* (and the PNP on which it's based) makes it easy for the healthcare provider to offer a "diet/nutrition prescription" for their patients. Simply, the PNP provides patients with an understanding of how their body processes the food they choose to eat, how it affects the pancreas, and the domino effect that poor choices have on their weight and their health. The PNP enables the patient to participate in their healing. No healthcare provider should bear the burden of healing any patient that continues to abuse themselves with wrong choices. The expectation that healthcare providers should be miracle workers who should have the power to reverse years of self-inflicted abuse is unfair. Patients must be educated on how to take responsibility for their health and should work alongside their healthcare provider to maximize modern medicine benefits and enhance their overall wellness.

The PNP will help the patient create a personalized plan for healthy eating. No "one size fits all" diet works. Bio-individuality is addressed in *The Pancreatic Oath*. Each body has three "voices" to express itself. Like it or not, these voices speak the truth. How your body looks naked, how much your body weighs, and how your blood glucose is affected by what you eat and drink—they all communicate how well or how poorly you are taking care of yourself. In order to succeed on the PNP, one must come to terms with these sometimes harsh realities:

1. The mirror doesn't lie.
2. The scale doesn't lie.
3. The glucometer doesn't lie.

As clinicians, it is crucial we make our own health a priority and model healthy behaviors to those we serve. Thus, I invite you to personally try the PNP and follow the protocol advocated in *The Pancreatic Oath*. It can help put your loved ones and your patients on the path to healthier eating that will lead to weight loss, improved blood work, reduction in medication, and an enhanced quality of life.

Please join me in protecting the pancreas. I look forward to assisting you in the delivery of this highly effective regimen. Please e-mail me at info@pnprogram.com about your success in using the PNP approach with your own patients.

At www.ILOVEMYPANCREAS.com, your patients can access the HIPAA compliant online nutrition journal we have provided in order to ensure the best results and safely track individual progress on the Pancreatic Nutritional Program.

Your First Assignment

1. Go to the full-length mirror in your house.
2. Lock the doors to the room.
3. Take off all your clothes.
4. Examine your naked body in the mirror.

What do you see? What is your body trying to tell you?

Like a detective, comb your body visually for evidence of what conditions it is trying to alert you to. Look for outward manifestations of what is occurring internally.

Look at your stomach, your thighs, your butt, your face, upper arms, etc. What do they tell you?

Are there bulges in all the wrong places? Blatant obesity? Or even just a bloated appearance to your face? Double chin? Triple chin? Cystic acne? Wounds that are slow to heal or have left scars? Do you have skin tags or skin discoloration? Do you have to lift skin to wash? Do you have excessive unwanted hair or increased hair growth? Circles under your eyes?

This is not meant to induce shame—it is meant to begin a dialogue with your body. The mirror is one of the three voices your body has to speak to you. If your body looks "abused" in anyway, it is time for you to listen to it and help it. You can help stop the abuse by eating wisely and exercising. Your body is alerting you to the damage you are causing to your health through your current consumption habits. You must respond to its messages if you are going to get in shape and feel better.

Please join me in protecting your pancreas,
a fundamental necessity for a future of
improved health and weight loss.
— Candice Rosen

CHAPTER ONE

Why the Pancreas? My Story

Why the Pancreas?

THE QUESTION "WHY THE PANCREAS?" has been answered for me in a very personal way. My daughter Jennifer was diagnosed with polycystic ovarian syndrome (PCOS) and pre-diabetes in her early 20s. Although she did not have all of the typical symptoms of a young woman with PCOS, she did struggle with cystic acne and weight gain. Her pre-diabetic symptoms were really those of insulin resistance.

Because she was young to be struggling with these issues, I took Jennifer to a variety of specialists, from gynecologists and dermatologists to registered dieticians, in order to discover the cause and cure for her condition. We sought the advice of an endocrinologist, a diabetes specialist. This consultation was unsatisfying, to say the least. The endocrinologist, like the other specialists, was essentially committing Jennifer to a life sentence of medication and no hope of escaping a life-long disease. Jennifer was given three prescriptions.

We declined the medications. Addressing the symptoms with medications that lead to serious side effects and not dealing with the source of Jennifer's condition was unacceptable. As someone who had a career in the medical field as a nurse and then social worker, I felt sickened by a trend in healthcare that I saw growing year after year. It seemed to me that American physicians have become "pharmaceutical bartenders," if you will, and their patients have been over-served for far too long!

> *Type 2 Diabetes is a*
> *CONSEQUENCE,*
> *not a DISEASE!*

I did not accept the fact that my daughter had an incurable illness. I felt that it was time to tackle the root cause of the disease, not mask it. Since we did not receive an acceptable treatment strategy from my daughter's endocrinologist, I was determined to find a solution that would have long-term benefits to her overall health.

There Must Be Something Else

I am a nurse trained in modern science and medicine. I did not spurn the knowledge that I was taught nor abandon the skills I have amassed for an untested treatment. Jennifer and I began with the accepted professional recommendations. We began following the American Diabetic Association (ADA) Diet faithfully. However, it soon became clear that counting carbohydrates and making the provided recipes was not working. There had to be something more, something better.

I decided that I was going to test my blood along with Jennifer. Each time she was required to prick her finger, place a drop of blood on a test strip that was inserted in a glucometer, and receive a blood sugar reading—I did the same. It soon became apparent that even though we were eating the same diet, it affected our blood glucose differently. A given meal might keep my blood sugar stable and cause Jennifer's blood sugar to spike and vice versa. Some meals Jennifer could handle and I couldn't; however, the majority of the time Jennifer showed a greater sensitivity. The only explanation for this was that Jennifer's pancreas was reacting differently than my pancreas to the same food.

I immediately realized that some of the American Diabetic Association recommendations do not work for every individual; clearly, *one size does not fit all*. For Jennifer and me, it was nothing less than amazing! Discovering what foods and food combinations (discussed in Chapter 9) raised blood glucose levels to an unhealthy state continues to be fascinating. In fact, Jennifer and I were so curious about how our bodies would process what we ate for breakfast, lunch, and dinner that we began betting on what our blood glucose numbers would be after certain meals.

After only five weeks of testing (and eating to protect the pancreas), Jennifer lost 26 pounds and I lost seven. I eventually went on to lose over 30 pounds and have kept it off, lowering my total cholesterol and triglycerides. My LDL (bad cholesterol) fell and my HDL (good cholesterol) increased. Jennifer not only lost weight, but her skin cleared up. Jennifer now understands what foods trigger her pancreas to overwork, and I understand what foods specifically affect mine.

But, of course, we are human. Jennifer and I do not always give the pancreas the respect it deserves. It can be easy to veer off the highway of pancreatic health if you give in to your cravings. Change is difficult. The difference for Jennifer and me is that we have the knowledge of *Self-Health* and we understand how to use it. When Jennifer goes off the path, she sees the negative results almost immediately—in her skin, sleep patterns, menstrual cycle, and her weight. These negatives help guide her back on the road to optimal wellness. The important point, however, is that she now has a long-term solution that works without medication. She is a happier and healthier individual having a deeper understanding of just how her body works.

The Pancreas and Health

Our journey provided us with a better understanding and appreciation for the critical role the pancreas plays in one's health. From weight gain to diabetes to heart disease, what you eat and how that food affects the pancreas has a direct effect on your health. It can cause or prevent future disease. It can cause you to gain or lose weight. This in itself is not a new concept. The real problem lies in the integration of knowledge and lifestyle practices. How many healthcare providers do you know that are overweight and out of shape? If they cannot get it together, how do they expect their patients to tackle the problem? Nutritional prescriptions are rarely written. The inability to explain the effect of poor food choices on the body as a whole is crippling our healthcare system. A simple understanding of how food choices impact your body and your health is very powerful knowledge indeed.

Without meaning to, a few years after my own amazing discovery with Jennifer, I was forced to test my theory again on myself. I have to admit that I became lazy and did not regularly choose my foods wisely. I did not eat to protect my pancreas. I gained weight. Then, an onslaught of serious health struggles prompted me to recommit myself to protecting my pancreas. During a routine exam, my gynecologist discovered a mass on my right ovary. Ovarian cancer (Stage I or Stage II) was suspected. I met with a gynecological surgical oncologist and prepared for the worst. I awoke from anesthesia to find out that the bizarre growth was benign. Although it had wrapped itself around my descending artery and ureter from my kidney to my bladder, I did *not* have cancer. What I *did have* was a blessing and another chance.

While the tumor was not malignant, it did need to be removed. This meant a total hysterectomy in which my uterus and ovaries were removed. The moment I no longer had ovaries I entered menopause, which left me with terrible hot flashes. With the cardiovascular protecting effects of estrogen now gone, my cholesterol levels slowly and steadily increased. In addition, I had no energy and I felt like crap.

Shortly thereafter, I began to routinely test my blood and discovered that my glucose levels were again way out of line. I was abusing my pancreas and jeopardizing my present and future health. The pancreatic abuse manifested itself in abnormal blood work: increasing cholesterol and blood glucose levels, but also things I could directly see and feel like weight gain and lethargy. Knowing my family's medical history, I knew that the genetic cards were stacked against me. If I could at all help it, I did not want to follow in their footsteps. In 2001, my dear mother, Nada, died from complications of pancreatic abuse that lead to diabetes. Like her brother, sisters, and her own mother and father, Nada suffered from the complications of diabetes: heart disease, stroke, kidney failure, diabetic retinopathy (blindness from diabetes), and vascular problems (that led to amputation of both legs for one sister). The complications of diabetes not only compromised their quality of life, but it also shortened their lives, robbing them of precious time.

I knew I had to make additional changes to protect myself from the medical baggage that my family carried. That meant I could no longer continue with my current way of eating. My husband, Steven, is also haunted by a family health history of heart disease and cancer. His increasing cholesterol level and his desire to lose weight prompted him to protect his pancreas, as well. Steven and I also did not want to be a burden to our children. Dealing with a parent (or parents) who suffers from a *self-inflicted* chronic illness is completely unfair.

After surgery, my total cholesterol, triglycerides, and LDL (bad cholesterol) numbers were high. The knee-jerk reaction in the healthcare industry is to prescribe drugs, but I did not want to become dependent on statin drugs—or any medication, if I could avoid it. My blood work showed a total cholesterol of 245, triglycerides of 56, LDL of 149, and HDL of 85. Are these the worst lipid levels ever? No. Do they warrant some sort of treatment? Absolutely. They were bad enough that, given my family history, my physician wanted to prescribe Lipitor. Just in case you have not heard of Lipitor, it is one of a class of drugs known as statins that work in the liver to improve blood cholesterol levels.

> *It is time to take control of your health, present and future. It is time to nurture your body, not poison it. What you eat affects your physical and mental health—remember that! There are NO simple solutions, i.e. a pill or gastric bypass. There are no quick fixes. Your health is YOUR responsibility, not your healthcare provider's.*

In addition to the Lipitor, I was prescribed Boniva (a calcium supplement), Effexor (to reduce hot flashes and help with possible depression; how could I be depressed when I found out that I did not have cancer?), and hormone replacement therapy. I refused ALL of it.

Help came from my daughter Melissa, a gifted writer, poet, and nutrition counselor. She and her husband, Greg Horos, are the creative owners of *LOCALI,* their conscious convenience store in Los Angeles, California. I am extremely proud of their commitment to sustainability, the green movement, and the belief that "food on the go," or "fast food," can and should be healthy.

Melissa convinced me to combine foods in a different way and to focus more on a plant-based protein "diet." She introduced me to an incredible book, *The China Study,* written by Dr. T. Colin Campbell. Doctor Campbell is the Jacob Gould Schurman Professor Emeritus of Nutritional Biochemistry at Cornell University and the Project Director of the China Oxford-Cornell Diet and Health Project. He is a revolutionary and has devoted over 40 years to nutrition research, courageously promoting improved health through a plant-based protein diet. *The China Study* is the most comprehensive study of health and nutrition ever conducted. Doctor Campbell's message is clear; however, for many companies in the food and healthcare industries, the ramifications of healthier eating have an adverse effect on their revenues. His is a powerful book on so many levels. His passion for educating the public about his research inspired me to start writing a book about the success I was having with my nutrition theory. As I wrote, my practice expanded from family and friends to a constant stream of clients arriving in my office completely by word of mouth.

I went on to become certified as a health counselor by the Institute for Integrative Nutrition, in order to learn how my program compared to other dietary theories from around the world. I became more confident that my simple, yet innovative approach was actually the best UN-DIET, since your body curates what you eat, rather than you forcing a particular set of dietary parameters on your body.

My original weight fluctuated between 145 and 158 pounds. I went back to the drawing board and reduced the amount of animal protein I consumed and altered my combination of foods. After three months, I weighed 129. My blood tests showed a significant improvement. My total cholesterol was 211—down from 245; LDL—115 (down from 149); HDL—88 (up from 85); triglycerides—41; and fasting glucose—85. My weight now fluctuates between 123 and 126. Can you appreciate the difference? These are the tracking numbers of good or bad health, and I managed to change them through good nutrition that was pancreatic friendly.

	Before PNP	**After PNP**
Body Weight	145–156 lbs	123–126 lbs
Total Cholesterol	245 mg/dl	211 mg/dl
LDL ("Bad cholesterol")	149 mg/dl	115 mg/dl
HDL ("Good cholesterol")	85 mg/dl	88 mg/dl
Triglycerides	56 mg/dl	41 mg/dl
Fasting Blood Glucose	92 mg/dl	85 mg/dl

Once again, I will admit to being human. Occasionally, I slip up; however, you can be sure my pancreas and my body let me know when I need to pay better attention. My body speaks to me either through my appearance (the mirror), weight gain (the scale), or higher than healthy blood glucose readings (the glucometer). The three voices of the body that never lie: (1) the mirror doesn't lie, (2) the scale doesn't lie, and (3) the glucometer doesn't lie. These little wake-up calls are enough for me to immediately return to the practice of *protecting my pancreas*. My concern for my pancreas and future health issues continues to outweigh the short-term pleasures of any processed food or sweet treat. My hope is that you will feel the same. By placing your pancreas in "idle mode," your cravings will decrease because you will not have the fluctuations in blood sugar that cause them.

The PNP is a way of life, not a diet. Your body is a living miracle. Your lungs never forget to take a breath. Your heart beats with precise regularity. Your body is not a garbage can for you to pollute with junk foods. If you treat it like one, then you should expect the consequences of such actions. On the other hand, if you provide your body with the tools that it needs like healthy, organic, pancreatic friendly foods, it will do all the work. Protecting your pancreas requires a lifestyle change. Are you up for it?

Change is hard. It requires work and an alteration in attitude. There is **NO** magic pill that can achieve *healthy* weight loss. Bariatric surgery does not remove **YOU** from the equation. Your body and your health are **YOUR** responsibility. Your eating habits, your attitude, and your behavior must change. You can do it! Jennifer, Steven, my clients, and I have reversed potential serious health issues by monitoring what we eat, checking our blood glucose, and respecting the pancreas. I invite you to practice *Self-Health* by taking responsibility for your body and its well-being.

An overworked pancreas leads to illness, decreased quality of life, and premature death. You can bank on it.

CHAPTER TWO

What is a Pancreas and What Does it Do?

"Science may have found a cure for most evils;
but it has found no remedy for the worst of them
all—the apathy of human beings."
—*Helen Keller*

THE PANCREAS IS THE fine-tuned engine that is an essential component of your digestive system. The pancreas makes digestive juices that facilitate the absorption of the food you have eaten. It is a light pinkish, soft and long, irregularly shaped gland (reminds me of a boomerang) that is located to the right of the spleen and behind the stomach.

In an adult, the pancreas is between 15 and 25 centimeters long (between 5.9 inches and 9.8 inches) and weighs

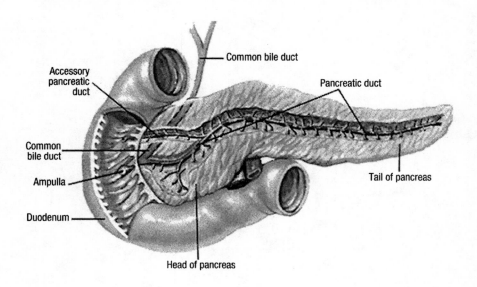

Accessory pancreatic duct

Common bile duct

Pancreatic duct

Common bile duct

Ampulla

Duodenum

Tail of pancreas

Head of pancreas

60–150 grams (between slightly over 2 ounces and slightly less than 5 ounces).

The function of the pancreas and its role in disease, especially diabetes, has not always been clear. The disease that we now call diabetes has been around for millennia. Ancient Greeks were the first to describe the diabetes disease: dia (through) + bainein (go/passer-through). They labeled it this way because those suffering from the disease urinated often and in large amounts. Although those early Greek physicians identified the symptoms of diabetes, they did not understand why the body produced excess urine.

The relationship between the pancreas and the disease of diabetes was shown in 1889 through the experiments of a German physician, Joseph von Mering, and his Lithuanian colleague, Dr. Oskar Minkowski. The two physicians figured out that the pancreas contains regulators that control blood sugar. It would take several more years to isolate those regulators as insulin and glucagon. Crystallized insulin was introduced in 1922, and commercial insulin, initially extracted from cows and pigs, was developed in 1927. The availability of an insulin replacement was an answered prayer for many who suffered from diabetes' symptoms and had no treatment options.

That is what the organ is, but what exactly does the pancreas do? Simply put, the pancreas produces and secretes hormones and enzymes that help the body digest and process the food that we eat. All cells of the body need sugar to fuel their processes, sort of like gas in a car. Without fuel, the car will not move. Without sugar, the cells will not function. It is our cells that are responsible for basically everything that we do. Our muscle cells move our limbs or pump our blood. Our nerve cells allow us to think and sense our surroundings. Our kidney cells filter our blood. Nothing gets done in the body, really, without a steady supply of sugar.

The pancreas secretes hormones and enzymes into the blood (endocrine function) or into the gastrointestinal tract (exocrine function). The pancreas' endocrine job is to produce insulin and glucagon. These hormones are released in response to meals and regulate sugar levels in the blood. Insulin is required to transfer molecules of sugar from the blood to the inside of cells throughout the body. Insulin acts like a key that opens the cell's door for sugar to enter. Without insulin to bind to the cell's "lock," sugar will not be able to get inside muscle, liver, or fat cells.

Glucagon, on the other hand, is a hormone that raises the level of glucose in the blood. Our bodies evolved to compensate for our historically inconsistent food supply. In the time of early man, periods of famine were commonplace. Today, it may be a full day of meetings, an international plane trip, or running to catch a train. The cells still need a steady supply of sugar, so glucagon stimulates the liver to release individual glucose links. These glucose (sugar) molecules are stored in long chains called glycogen. When glucagon is released by the pancreas, the liver starts cutting off individual glucose links (molecules) from that long chain of glycogen.

Every time you put something in your mouth (a liquid or solid food) — please pause and ask yourself, "WILL MY PANCREAS HAVE TO WORK HARD?" or "IS THIS BAD FOR MY PANCREAS?" If your answer is YES to either question, then DO NOT eat it.

Neither insulin nor glucagon aids in digestion; however, the pancreas does aid in digestion. The pancreas' exocrine function is to produce bicarbonate and digestive enzymes. Both bicarbonate and insulin are released into the lumen of the small intestine by way of the pancreatic duct. Since the stomach produces an intensely acidic environment, food moving from the stomach to the intestine needs to be neutralized. Bicarbonate works to create a neutral pH in the first part of the small intestine (duodenum). This neutral pH protects the intestine from acid damage, but also creates an environment that allows other pancreatic enzymes to do their thing. Digestive enzymes released from the pancreas help break down large bits of food into small molecules that can be easily transferred in the blood and processed by cells.

The role of the pancreas in digestion begins the moment you put food into your mouth. Let's say you take a bite of pizza. As you chew, salivary glands in your mouth excrete saliva in order to break down the pizza. Saliva contains amylase. Amylase is an enzyme that aids in the digestion of starch. When you swallow the pizza, it travels down your esophagus into your stomach. From there it goes to the small intestines where the pizza is broken down even further into basic fats, carbohydrates, proteins, and glucose (the metabolized form of sugar). The digestive enzymes from the pancreas and liver are released through ducts into the small intestine. At this point, digestion becomes interesting. What you have eaten can either be good or bad for your pancreas (and you). When it is bad, it is abuse.

CHAPTER THREE

Pancreas Abuse

> "A wise man should consider that health is
> the greatest of human blessings."
> —*Hippocrates*

Sugar, Sugar Everywhere

THE PANCREAS REACTS TO whatever you eat. Let's begin with the category of sugar. The foods that fall under this heading are often surprising to people. They believe sugar includes a piece of cake, pie, or candy; however, they are surprised to learn that white flour pasta, white bread, starchy vegetables, processed foods, or unhealthy refined carbohydrates are quickly and directly converted into small sugar molecules by the stomach and intestines. Even if you are not eating pie and candy, you are still getting a lot of sugar.

Sugar molecules (glucose) cross intestinal membranes and are absorbed into the blood. Glucose is then carried through the bloodstream either to be used by the cells of the body or to be stored. If you eat the wrong food for you in large amounts, combine foods improperly and lead a sedentary lifestyle, then the food (fuel/glucose) is stored. In the liver, it is stored as glycogen (for emergency energy). In the body, it is stored as fat. Your body can grow (every which way) in order to accommodate the excess food consumption (as showcased in the obesity epidemic); however, your liver has limited storage capacity. When the liver reaches its limit on storing glycogen, the glycogen is converted into triglycerides and released in your bloodstream. Perhaps you have heard of triglycerides as one of the cholesterol markers that physicians check when they order a lipid panel (along with LDL, HDL, and total cholesterol). This is the link between an abused pancreas, high cholesterol numbers, and heart disease. It is a domino effect triggered and driven by repeated bad food choices.

> *You have heard the phrase "You are what you eat." Your health depends on what you eat.*

If you are a fairly active individual, the good news is that 50% of what you have eaten is used for immediate energy; however, if you are a couch potato and spend too much time sitting or lying around, the news is not good. Only 10% is stored in the muscle and liver in the form of glycogen, while 40% is converted into and stored as fats, triglycerides, and cholesterol. That is bad news for those who overwork their pancreas with poor food choices. Obesity and heart disease become health issues.

The domino effect I spoke about earlier becomes even more serious when we look at what high glucose levels cause: high levels of insulin. Insulin is inflammatory, toxic to the lining of your veins, arteries, and capillaries. Can you imagine the long-term effects of high levels of glucose and insulin circulating throughout your body and bathing your vital organs in a toxic environment of your own making?

Think about all that you eat in a given day. What do you think happens to that 50% if it isn't used for immediate energy? If you don't exercise or haven't had to lift a car off of someone (example of using your adrenaline and glycogen supplies), your unhealthy eating habits add up. They are showcased by your obvious holding tanks: your stomach, your thighs, your butt, your face, your upper arms. It isn't pretty and it certainly isn't healthy!

Food Choices and Health

What you eat, *your* food choices, have a direct effect on the health of every organ in *your* body. Poor food choices and a sedentary lifestyle lead to illness and the slow destruction of your body. High sugar and refined carbohydrate diets, stress, and lack of exercise can generate elevated glucose levels in both blood and tissue.[1] The way to ensure improved health is to keep your pancreas in idle mode. Your pancreas should be on call, not working overtime. The load it pulls should be in keeping with its capacity as a fine-tuned machine. In other words, be careful what you ingest or you are headed for a health breakdown.

Most Americans unknowingly abuse their pancreas on a daily basis and the consequences can be devastating. The average American diet includes about 40% to 50% carbohydrates.[2] According to the U.S. Department of Agriculture's Continuing Survey of Food Intakes by Individuals (CSFII), the average U.S. adult consumes 20 teaspoons of added sugar each day. If you consume too many sugars, your poor, exhausted pancreas has to pump out massive amounts of insulin to deal with the overload. Because it takes vitamins and minerals to process the carbohydrates, B vitamins and chromium are depleted, among others. This can lead to low energy and additional side effects from increasing nutrient deficiencies related to pancreatic abuse.

> *Processed food pollutes your body and destroys your health. It also creates a dependency on the healthcare system.*

When you overload your body with a poor food choice, the rising levels of sugar in your blood strain your pancreas. Thus, large meals make the pancreas work very hard to deliver the needed insulin. Eventually, after years of being overworked through poor diet, the pancreas cannot meet the demand. Diets that are high in simple and refined sugars and fats, and low in complex carbohydrates result in diabetes, high blood pressure, kidney disease, heart disease, and some cancers.[3]

An Overworked Pancreas

I believe overworking the pancreas leads to insulin overproduction. In turn, insulin overproduction burns out the pancreas and eventually leads to full-blown diabetes. The pancreas was never "built" to be a workhorse for *overconsumption* or to keep up with the workload imposed upon it by eating massive quantities of unhealthy food. Imagine a compact, fine-tuned sports car trying to pull a fully loaded semi-trailer up a very steep hill. No matter how hard the high-performance car might strain, it simply will not get that load up the hill without damaging the engine. Obviously, this is not a reasonable way to handle the sports car; it is, in fact, abusive to the engine and the powertrain of an otherwise powerful vehicle. It does not take a mechanic to know that the result of that behavior will be a breakdown. Likewise, it does not take a health-care professional to see that abusing the pancreas will eventually destroy it.

The goal of *The Pancreatic Oath* and the Pancreatic Nutritional Program (PNP)™ is to protect the pancreas. This, in turn, will increase your quality of life, by preventing, stabilizing or reversing chronic illnesses related to diet. A calendar filled with doctor's appointments is a compromised life. Don't destroy your body and your health by burning out your pancreas.

Wisely choosing what you put in your mouth and increasing your metabolism through activity and exercise are easier than you might think. You can do it once you understand what your pancreas likes and does not like.

Listen to your pancreas and your body—they will guide you to improved health.

It is up to you. You have to care enough about yourself and your future health. Believe me, IT IS WORTH IT.

Change is difficult. I understand; however, poor choices and living to eat instead of eating to live will affect your weight, your health, and your quality of life.

Remember:

The food you choose to eat has a direct effect on your pancreas. Bad choices will cause weight gain and health issues.

Pancreas Abuse

The Pancreatic Oath definition of pancreatic abuse:

When the intake of poor food choices and/or the overconsumption of food outweigh or exceed the capability of the pancreas.

CHAPTER FOUR

The Signs of an Abused Pancreas and an Abusive Healthcare System

> "Health is not valued till sickness comes."
> — *Dr. Thomas Fuller*

A S THE FORMER DIRECTOR of Gilda's Club Chicago, a cancer support center for men, women, children, and their family and friends, I empathized with many cancer patients who felt they "stood out" because of treatment side effects. They would complain that their hair loss and pale skin drew attention to their health issues. Wigs, creative scarves, and make-up were used in order to avoid wearing their diagnoses on their sleeve, so to speak.

It was heart wrenching to hear story after story of cancer patients who felt blindsided by their cancer diagnosis. They would ask, "How did it happen? Could I have prevented this cancer?" Unless they had spent years smoking or working in a toxic environment, most patients had no idea how they "got cancer." Although hereditary factors are a risk for developing cancer (a strong risk in some), environmental factors, nutrition, and lifestyle choices have an important effect.[4]

Well, people who abuse their pancreas wear their "illness" on their sleeve, too. Metabolic syndrome, insulin resistance, pre-diabetes, and polycystic ovarian syndrome are several conditions that are obvious and characterized by obesity, abnormal hair growth (hirsutism), cystic acne, bloated (pincushion) appearance, poor wound healing, and a flushed face.

When they ask, "How did this happen?" the answer is simple: eating the wrong foods, drinking the wrong beverages, lack of portion control and exercise.

Pancreas Abuse as the Cause of Disease

I believe pancreatic abuse is a major risk factor for the development of chronic diseases—heart disease, stroke, high blood pressure, high cholesterol, vascular problems, kidney problems, visual problems, pre-diabetes, insulin resistance, metabolic syndrome, polycystic ovarian syndrome, and diabetes. It is not a mystery. Preventing these diseases is certainly a better choice than dealing with the consequences after they have occurred.

Consider which is preferable: (A) taking steps that require self-control and exercise to prevent a disease, or (B) being committed to taking prescribed medications every day for the rest of your life, living with pain and sickness, and/or worst case—undergoing surgeries like cardiac bypass surgery, amputation, or stomach stapling?

Unfortunately, modern medicine is focused on putting out fires after they are ablaze rather than preventing the fire in the first place. This is why many people leave their doctor's office with a prescription rather than knowledge on how to take charge of their own health.

> *Respect your body. Physicians and medication are not just THE answer. You have a responsibility to work in conjunction with your physician to improve and maintain your health. Start with what you put in your mouth.*

We don't have much control in life, but we do have control over what we put in our mouths. What effect it will have on our bodies depends on whether what we eat is good or bad for our pancreas. Whether it's food, drugs, or alcohol—whatever isn't good for the pancreas will end up costing us in the long run. That double cheeseburger, fries, super-sized soft drink, or six-pack of beer may taste great for the moment—but you will pay dearly for those moments of pleasure. There is no way around it—poor choices equal poor health.

Of course, the damage that we do to our bodies through poor food choices isn't always immediately apparent. When we are young, we can more or less eat what we want and feel no ill effects. Eat a double cheeseburger and the body simply processes it. The sugar, fat, and protein is broken down and converted into energy. Even when you are young, your pancreas strains at this burden. If you were riding in a fine-tuned sports car, you would hear the engine strain at the extra workload. Unfortunately, the pancreas is silent and overlooked; yet it struggles with this food burden all the same.

You Are HOW You Eat

The pancreas' cry for help becomes obvious in a person's weight and appearance. The bloated, full-moon look of the face, torso shaped a like barrel, heavy thighs, double/triple chin, and so on. These individuals appear puffy—like a human pincushion—they are FAT. Look around, look in the mirror—do you look like that? Do any of your children or loved ones look like that? Do you purchase clothing in sizes like XXXL? Do you feel uncomfortable in an airplane coach seat? These questions are the beginning of an honest dialogue to determine—Are you abusing your pancreas?

> *Remember, you can be thin and still abuse your pancreas.*

Read this carefully:

It is *not just* the weight.

It is what the weight represents: Pancreatic Abuse and Poor Health.

Food, either too much or the wrong kind, will eventually destroy your life. I was recently at a restaurant with my 88-year-old father, when a family of three entered the dining area. The mother, father, and their son were huge. They could barely walk. They huffed and puffed their way to a table and proceeded to order their food. Not surprisingly, they made terrible choices in large amounts. My father just shook his head and said, "I'd rather walk than eat." Individuals that would rather *eat* than *walk* live for today, not tomorrow. Their slow suicide via unhealthy food is painful to witness.

You Eat What You Have Been Told To

In our world of mass communication and limitless information, people still do not know how to nourish their precious bodies. They lack the necessary information and self-awareness. They don't know that their unhealthy eating habits have gone "too far," until they are diagnosed with a chronic illness. Even then, they are reluctant to change their eating habits because now treatment comes in a pill or a shot.

Finding one excuse after another, their mindset comes not from within, but from out there, in the form of print ads and television commercials urging them to consume everything and anything. With no thought for tomorrow, the consuming public is assaulted by print, Internet, and television commercials. They are victims of corporations, marketing companies, and advertisers. There are Surgeon General warning labels on packs of cigarettes. Why not a heart attack, diabetes, or stroke warning on the side of certain food packages and fast food menus? Will any of the major food corporations send a representative to sit with you while you undergo renal dialysis? Or help you recover from open-heart surgery? Will they pay for a portion of your monthly medications not covered by insurance? Of course, not. They will claim that, as an educated, sophisticated consumer, you should have known the risks. But where are you to become educated? From advertising and marketing gurus?

Many corporate entities profit from an intertwined relationship among processed food manufacturers and the ever-expanding healthcare business. Our healthcare industry has been bulking up alongside the food industry for far too long. It has become more and more acceptable to expect the patient to tell the doctor what he or she needs. We seem to be living in a society that believes your health, your life, is not your responsibility. In fact, your only responsibility is to consume. Your health has become your physician's responsibility. It is presumed your physician will take care of whatever health problems arise—that's his or her job. Not *your* job. Again, your job is to consume. That is the message pushed by the pharmaceutical companies, media, and advertisers.

Drugs for all types of ailments are marketed and promoted on television, on the Internet, and in print—even on theater playbills. Patients are indoctrinated to ask for medicines they have been told *they need* by pharmaceutical companies. You never see a commercial about how your pancreas is being abused by your behavior, but you see dozens of commercials for medicines to treat diabetes once it occurs. Can't sleep—ask your physician for Sleepinol; can't relax—ask your physician for Relaxinate; can't get an erection—ask your physician for Erectra. Patients tell their physicians what they want or think they need because they saw it on television. They live as abusively as they want, relying on the miracle of modern medicine to be their safety net. Patients have relinquished their personal responsibility over their health and their health is suffering in the process.

Over the past decade or two, there has been what I believe to be a dangerous shift in the way healthcare is delivered. Today's physician is no longer the "teacher" educating his or her patients on disease prevention via good nutrition, exercise, and personal habits. The physician's goal is to "fix it" rather than "prevent it." Typical patient thinking goes like this: the physician will prescribe something—gastric bypass, cholesterol-lowering drugs, the insulin pump, blood pressure medication, renal dialysis, or a cardiac

> *Diabetes is a gold mine. The food industry preys upon the uneducated consumer. It has made the industry wealthy and cost Americans their health and quality of life.*

bypass. In other words, the physician will clean up the mess, a "patch job" until the next health crisis. Yet the underlying cause, years of abuse via diet and lifestyle choices, was never adequately addressed when it could have had an impact on health.

The onslaught of managed care and escalating health-care costs mean that now it is more important than ever to take care of your own health by protecting your pancreas. The idea of *Self-Health* is an idea whose time has come. The concept is especially timely now since we face constant changes in the politics and legislation of healthcare insurance. This state of flux in healthcare coverage is a major reason for each and every one of us to focus on what we can do to help ourselves. You will benefit financially and physically by taking your consumption habits seriously.

The Decision is Yours

If you don't care about your health and your future health, if you don't mind being a prisoner of your body and its deterioration, then by all means continue to abuse your pancreas. If cheeseburgers, fries, and soft drinks are worth obesity, polycystic ovarian syndrome, metabolic syndrome, insulin resistance, diabetes, cardiovascular illness, stroke, and kidney failure, then eat and drink up!

Good health is a blessing and should not be taken for granted. It is my wish that you do not allow yourself or your loved ones to be victims of processed food companies, Big Pharma, and their advertisers. The key to *Self-Health* is in understanding how the body works, how the pancreas works, and how the food we eat affects our health and well-being. Doctors and hospitals can no longer shoulder all of the responsibility for correcting the gluttony and poor choices that have driven the health of millions of Americans to a diabetes epidemic. We need to unlearn the bad information, block out the propaganda and the advertisements, and make the commitment to live a life of health starting today.

Clearly, you must take responsibility for your own good health. You SHOULD exercise control over what you purchase and what you consume. That responsibility does not end with you—it extends to loved ones, friends, and our society at large. You must exercise that responsibility and spread the word about protecting the pancreas.

Think of it this way—there is no processed food that is worth destroying your health. There is no snack or junk food worth destroying the well-being and good health of a child. I believe it is time for our entire society to get a grip, get over the gluttony and instant gratification, and refuse to be enslaved by major food corporations and pharmaceutical companies.

How?

Start by focusing on healing your pancreas and your body.

An Example of Change

Before she began the Pancreatic Nutritional Program (PNP), one of my clients, Francine (*name changed to protect privacy*) had told me that her "mouth had a party at every meal and snack." Well, all that changed for her following the PNP. Francine lost 83 pounds on the program and wants to lose 30 more before her son's wedding. Having been on almost every other weight loss program (losing no more than 30 pounds and gaining back the 30 and more every time), Francine had yo-yoed her entire adult life. Francine never understood how her body processed food, nor the role the pancreas played in her weight and health issues. Equipped with knowledge, the "mouth party" was no longer an everyday binge fest. Francine is living the life she was meant to live. Her vibrant vitality feels better than any food could ever taste. She exercises, is off all medication (when she started, she was taking medicine for her blood pressure and a statin for her cholesterol), sleeps better and looks fantastic!

The PNP is for those individuals who have spent their lives "dieting" and exercising to lose weight instead of eating and exercising to prevent chronic illness and promote health. The PNP is also for those individuals interested in figuring out what their bodies need in order to heal. The PNP is for those individuals who, by changing the food they purchase, the way they prepare their food, and the way they eat—want to quietly (yet effectively) protest against big processed food corporations and factory farming. They want to stand up and become a voice for themselves, their loved ones, and their communities who believe healthy, naturally grown food is a consumer's right. They are part of a silent revolution that plays out in grocery stores, convenience stores, and restaurants (sit-down and drive-thru) every day. Their cause: health and well-being.

It is your duty every day as a citizen of the world to figure out how you can make a small difference in your health, the health of your family, and the health of your community. Ultimately, this collective cherishing of our natural resources and our bodies will have a positive ripple effect on the health of the planet.

Don't be Passive, be Proactive!

CHAPTER FIVE

Diabetes and the Pancreas

"Quit worrying about your health. It'll go away."
—Robert Orben

THE PANCREATIC OATH IS NOT a book about diabetes, nor is it a book solely for diabetics. However, I believe that a chapter dedicated to diabetes is important in the face of the worldwide epidemic of diabetes. When you consider how many people are ultimately diagnosed with diabetes and insulin resistance, it may be helpful to think of each healthy person as **pre-pre-diabetic**. You may not have diabetes now, but the risk of you developing the disease at some point in your life is disturbingly high. Understanding diabetes now, when you are a **pre-pre-diabetic**, is critical to perceiving the role of pancreatic abuse in the disease and preventing full-blown diabetes.

Diabetes mellitus is now an epidemic. Two hundred and forty-six million people have diabetes; 80% of them live in developing countries.[5] In fact, an estimated 24.1 million Americans have diabetes.[6] In addition, approximately 57 million Americans have pre-diabetes, a condition that may progress to clinical diabetes if not detected and treated in time.[7]

> *Juvenile diabetic patients—in particular those diagnosed under the age of five, are a blank slate. It is much easier to place them on the highway to good/ improved health than let's say a 13-year-old. No endocrinologist knows whether the Type 1 juvenile diabetic's pancreas is operating at 2%, 10%, or 25%. However, we can only hypothesize that once the diagnosis is made and the patient and his or her family begins "counting carbs" and relying on insulin— they will further destroy what little function is left of the pancreas and its ability to produce even a small amount of insulin.*

Those are alarming numbers.

Diabetes is a disease in which the body either does not produce insulin or the cells of the body cannot properly use insulin. Insulin is manufactured in the pancreas. The pancreas releases insulin in response to the foods that you consume. The cells of the body are designed to drink up all of the sugar that they can, but they must have insulin around to facilitate absorption of that sugar. If the insulin system does not work properly, the sugar will just stay in the blood vessels and eventually get excreted by the kidneys in the urine.

Glucose Needs Insulin

Why might this insulin system not work properly? Glucose needs to be present in the blood. It is what fuels the cells. The food that we eat is digested into small glucose (sugar) molecules and absorbed into the bloodstream.

Now that the sugar is in the bloodstream, it has to get into the cells of the body. Insulin has to be released by the pancreas, circulate in the blood, and bind to insulin receptors on cells. Insulin acts like a key that opens the cell's door to sugar entry. Without insulin to bind to the cell's "lock," sugar will not be able to get inside the way it needs to.

For people with Type 1 diabetes mellitus, the pancreas simply does not produce enough insulin to be released into the bloodstream. In people with this form of diabetes, insulin needs to be injected into the body to unlock the door. Without insulin injections, Type 1 diabetes can be rapidly fatal.

The problem is a little different in Type 2 diabetes mellitus. In this disease, the pancreas has the ability to make insulin. The problem is that the cells do not seem to recognize the "key" like it once did. Something changes in the "lock," if you will, that makes insulin less effective. Thus, a person eats a meal, sugar molecules travel through the bloodstream, both insulin and sugar reach the cells, but the cells more or less ignore the visitors. Sure, they will let some sugar inside, but they demand greater amounts of insulin to let in the same amount of sugar than they did before the disease.

In Type 2 diabetes, insulin injections are not always needed. For a while, doctors can manage the disease by giving oral medicines to artificially reduce the sugar burden on the body or trick the cells into accepting more sugar. Over time, the oral medicines are no longer effective in tricking the body and insulin injections are needed. The cells demand relatively monstrous doses of insulin to just accept the most modest amounts of sugar.

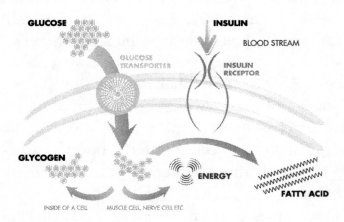

The Problem of Too Much Sugar in the Blood

So what if the cells do not accept the sugar? What is the big deal of letting the excess sugar/glucose stay in the bloodstream? The answer is that high levels of sugar in the blood are incredibly destructive. Over the short term, high levels of blood sugar, called hyperglycemia, can cause immediately life-threatening illnesses. If the blood sugar goes very high, it can lead to diabetic ketoacidosis or hyperosmolar hyperglycemia. These related conditions may cause temporary paralysis or problems with vision. They may cause drowsiness, delirium, and even coma. If the blood sugar is not lowered, the condition can be fatal.

Over the long term, hyperglycemia can ravage the eyes, kidneys, and nerves. High blood glucose/sugar can destroy the eye's retina and can ultimately lead to blindness. In the kidneys, diabetes affects blood filtration and the production of urine. Kidney damage might eventually force patients to have dialysis in order to simply filter their blood. The nerves hate high blood sugar. They stop working properly in a bath of high glucose levels, which leads to numbness and/or tingling, usually first in the feet, then the hands and chest.

High blood sugar affects wound healing, too. We take for granted the fact that small cuts and scrapes heal within a few days. In diabetics, this system does not function the way that it should. Small wounds may take weeks or more to heal. Consider an all too often scenario: A person with diabetes has decreased sensation in the feet because the high blood sugar has affected the nerves. That person can no longer feel certain objects

Once a diagnosis of diabetes is made, the body (the pancreas) should be placed on lockdown and only healthy, appropriate pancreatic "friendly" food should be ingested.

after stepping on them. The skin breaks or punctures, causing a wound. The wound cannot heal because high blood sugar interferes with the cells and proteins needed to close the wound. Now understand that humans are not the only species that need sugar to survive. Bacteria love sugar and will multiply rapidly in and on the skin of someone with diabetes—it is like a candy store for them. Thus, a simple wound becomes infected and takes even longer to heal, even with antibiotics.

According to The American Diabetic Association, the symptoms of diabetes are:

+ Frequent urination
+ Excessive thirst
+ Extreme hunger
+ Unusual weight loss
+ Increased fatigue
+ Irritability
+ Blurry vision

Why do diabetics lose weight or urinate in great amounts? Scientifically speaking, the "passing through of water/urine" occurs because the body's filtered load of glucose exceeds the ability of tubular re-absorption in the kidney. This inability to reabsorb glucose in the tubules results in diuresis (the secretion and passage of abnormally large amounts of urine). This water loss through urine leads to dehydration, which leads to thirst. In straightforward terms, too much sugar in the blood overwhelms the kidney's ability to process it. The kidney is designed to aggressively absorb sugar back into the bloodstream so that it does not pass into the urine. In fact, this state is sometimes referred to as glucose "spilling" into the urine to describe the state in which the sugar amount is so great that the kidneys cannot handle it. Until the 11th century, physicians of antiquity diagnosed diabetes by tasting the urine. In people with diabetes, the urine tastes sweet. The term "diabetes mellitus" roughly translates to "excessive sweet urine." I will take their word for it.

You may ask why it would be so bad to spill sugar in the urine. Isn't the problem too much sugar in the blood anyway? Unfortunately, when the sugar overwhelms the kidneys, it takes a lot of free water with it, too. This leads to dehydration, which is sometimes severe. If you have ever wondered why people with diabetes are excessively thirsty, this is a big reason why.

This constant dehydration leads to weight loss. Again, you may say, "But wait, I thought obesity leads to diabetes. Wouldn't it be better to weigh less?" While this may sound reasonable, you do not want to lose weight through dehydration, just like you do not want to lose weight through starvation.

In fact, some of the weight loss that occurs as a result of diabetes comes from a form of starvation. Since the cells do not accept glucose/sugar inside because of the reduced effects of insulin, they are starved of the sugar they need to survive. What we are left with is diabetes and its serious health consequences.

Type 1 Diabetes

According to the American Association of Clinical Endocrinologists, Type 1 diabetes "accounts for only five to ten percent of all diabetes cases. Type 1 diabetes is caused by an absolute deficiency of insulin secretion due to cellular-mediated autoimmune destruction of the pancreatic B-cells." The pancreas just isn't making insulin or enough of it. The cause? One appealing theory is that a viral insult is associated with the destruction of islet cells. Islet cells are the cell type that produces insulin in the pancreas. Many times, Type 1 diabetics have been diagnosed after a viral infection. The medical debate begins here: Endocrinologists are unable to determine the exact extent of pancreatic damage in Type 1 diabetes.

In determining how best to treat the ensuing diabetes, the question must be asked, "How can a pancreas that has suffered from a viral infection 'heal' when the patient adds insult to injury by ingesting food that raises the blood glucose level and forces a 'sick' pancreas to work overtime?" In essence, the pancreas continues to be "attacked" by what the body ingests. Insulin is prescribed and yet a proper diet that places the pancreas in "idle" mode in order to rest and heal is never prescribed. The diabetic patient continues to assault the pancreas with the wrong food by counting carbohydrates and taking injectable insulin.

I believe that once a diagnosis of diabetes (especially Type 1) is made, the body should be placed on a nutritional "lockdown," and only healthy, appropriate pancreatic "friendly" foods should be eaten. Carbohydrate counting is not always pancreatic friendly, as Jennifer and I discovered. This is a hypothesis that deserves testing.

The majority of diabetic patients are on a one-size-fits-all program of a carbohydrate counting diet and either insulin or oral medication. If the pancreas was placed on "lockdown," or "idle mode," in order to heal, the pancreatic function might improve. Instead of zero function, perhaps Type 1 diabetics could go on to have 20% function or 50% function of the pancreas, reducing their dosage of insulin or oral medications and improve their chances of avoiding the most severe consequences of diabetes.

An alternative theory advanced by Dr. T. Colin Campbell suggests the dangerous path toward Type 1 diabetes may begin at infancy. Studies have shown that babies and children reared on cow-based formula or cow's milk exhibit a higher incidence of Type 1 diabetes. According to the May 7, 2008 issue of *Science Daily*, researchers in Maine reported a new explanation for this mysterious link between consumption of cows' milk in infant formula early in life and an increased risk of later developing Type 1 diabetes. A protein in cow's milk appears to trigger an unusual immune response. The immune system recognizes the cow protein as foreign and tries to attack it. Unfortunately, the immune system apparently also erroneously attacks and destroys insulin-producing cells in the pancreas. In other words, the immune system confuses a protein on pancreatic islet cells with the protein in cow's milk.

Scientists do not fully understand the link between cow's milk and diabetes. They know, however, that beta-lactoglobulin, a protein present in cow's milk, but not found in human breast-milk or soy-based formula, is structurally similar to the human protein glycodelin, which controls the production of T-cells. T-cells help guard the body against infection. It is thought that an infant's immature immune system may inadvertently destroy glycodelin in an effort to destroy the similar cow's milk protein, which the system recognizes as foreign. It is a form of "friendly fire."

Type 2 Diabetes

The other form of diabetes—Type 2—now accounts for 90 to 95% of all diabetes cases. In this type of diabetes, the pancreas is able to produce insulin, but the body is unable to use it. According to the American Diabetic Association website, approximately 6.2 million Americans are undiagnosed Type 2 diabetics (this number does not include the 57 million diagnosed with pre-diabetes). Undiagnosed pancreatic abuse, along with this undetected clinical problem, leads to heart disease, stroke, high blood pressure, renal problems, and obesity.

The statistics surrounding Type 2 diabetes tell an equally disturbing story about the consequences of this epidemic for our society. For individuals born in the year 2000, the estimated lifetime risk for developing diabetes (Type 1 or Type 2) is 33% for males and 39% for females. The risk for death among individuals with diabetes is almost twice than of individuals without diabetes of similar age.[8]

Diabetes is a growing burden on those who suffer from it, their loved ones, and our entire society. Not only do high blood sugar levels create health problems, but also so do high insulin levels. When your pancreas is forced to produce more insulin, due to what you have eaten, the excess insulin (*remember the key that can no longer open the door to the cell*) results in inflammation of your cells and can have an adverse effect on your cardiovascular system.

Insulin and Insulin Resistance

Insulin resistance, which involves the inability of insulin to open the door to your cell, results in excess insulin circulating through your body. It may play a part in reduced levels of HDL (the good cholesterol), estrogen in women, or testosterone in men, while elevating bad cholesterol and triglyceride levels. The decrease in estrogen is exhibited in young women suffering from polycystic ovarian syndrome. Too much insulin has an effect on the production of estrogen, thus elevating testosterone levels. This explains the irregular periods, acne, and the hirsutism PCOS sufferers experience. Remember, research already links insulin resistance to high blood pressure, obesity, and Type 2 diabetes. Insulin resistance interferes with normal cholesterol function and fat storage (displayed in beer guts and metabolic syndrome).

High levels of insulin are toxic to the body, mainly by causing inflammation. Excess insulin has a destructive effect on your eyes. It can cause bleeding in the eye and lead to diabetic retinopathy (partial or total blindness).

Excess insulin also affects your kidneys, your heart, your brain, and the vessels in your body. Insulin at increased levels inflames the tissue. Continued inflammation can lead to irritation or, worse, ulceration—causing damage to the lining of an artery or vein.

The body attempts to repair this damage and, in doing so, creates a plaque, which is similar to a speed bump on a street. After years of pancreatic abuse due to unhealthy eating, the speed bumps become collecting areas for circulating cholesterol and fats (lipids) in your body. Cholesterol can move into the cell wall of arteries, restrict or reduce blood flow, and increase pressure in the artery (causing blood pressure issues). These speed bumps become breeding grounds for clot and plaque formation. If a particle breaks off, you'll be in trouble. The debris can travel to a vital organ in your body—brain, heart, or lungs—causing a catastrophic event.

> *It is YOUR body, not your physician's body or your spouse's or your friend's—it is your body and unless you want to spend your golden years like the vast majority of Americans—in poor health with their conversations saturated with what medication they are on and how high their cholesterol is—you must decide to change TODAY.*

Can you imagine what happens to your arteries and veins over the years from continual abuse due to the over-production of insulin caused by what you've been eating?

The vessels eventually narrow. It is much more difficult for blood to circulate properly and this narrowing places an extra burden on your heart, which has to pump much harder to get the blood through narrow (arteriosclerotic) arteries. This cycle of abuse results in high blood pressure, obstructed vessels, and a heart that is forced to work even harder to pump blood.

Diabetes and Obesity Are at Epidemic Proportions

Pancreatic abuse and resulting obesity are precursors to Type 2 diabetes, pre-diabetic syndrome, metabolic syndrome, insulin resistance, and polycystic ovarian syndrome. High blood glucose/sugar can damage the heart and blood vessels, kidneys, nerves, and eyes, and can cause disability and death from heart disease, stroke, kidney failure, amputations, and blindness.[9]

The years of pancreatic abuse will most likely result in chronic illness before you EVER receive a full-blown diagnosis of diabetes!

Diabetes and Cancer

Physicians have suspected the link between cancer and diabetes for years, but only recently have there been clinical studies to back it up. Doctors realized long ago that cancer and diabetes occur in the same patients much more often than they would if simply occurring by chance. When they carefully studied the issue, they found that diabetes increases the risk of liver cancer, pancreatic cancer, and cancer of the endometrium by 200%.[10] Other cancers such as breast, colon, and bladder cancers are increased by 20 to 50%.

Dr. Katherine A. McGlynn, a senior investigator at the United States National Cancer Institute, stated that control of diabetes might reduce the incidence of liver cancer. By using the SEER-Medicare linked database, researchers discovered that the leading cause of liver cancer was diabetes—an astonishing 33.5% of 5,600 people diagnosed with liver cancer had diabetes.

The prevalence of obesity among adults and children has risen significantly in the United States during the past 20 years. The latest data from the National Center for Health Statistics shows that more than 60 million Americans 20 years or older (30%) are obese. The percentage of young Americans who are overweight has more than tripled since 1980; approximately 9 million children, adolescents, and young adults 6 to 19 years of age (16%) are considered overweight.[11] These numbers represent millions of Americans who abuse their pancreases. The pancreas is unable to keep up with the demand placed upon it through eating the wrong way. When you consider the statistics surrounding obesity in our society and understand that this is the next step toward diabetes, and possibly cancer, protecting the pancreas becomes even more important.

While the biological link between cancer and diabetes is complex, one factor that links the diseases is elevated levels of insulin in the blood. Higher than normal insulin levels, called hyperinsulinemia, affect cancer cells in a number of unfortunate ways. Cancer cells have receptors on them that recognize insulin. The receptors are known as insulin-like growth factor or (IGF) receptors. As you may have guessed, when insulin binds to these receptors, cancer cells grow and flourish. There are other more complex ways that insulin can promote the growth of cancer cells, but the bottom line is that hyperinsulinemia—too much insulin in the blood—helps cancer cells grow. Cancer cells also love glucose.[12]

These facts are disturbing and alarming, yet they can be counteracted. By protecting your pancreas, you may prevent or postpone life-threatening illnesses. You can keep insulin and glucose levels right where they should be.

Diabetes—The Epidemic—The Facts

According to the International Diabetes Federation:

+ Diabetes affects 246 million people worldwide.
+ Diabetes will affect 380 million people by 2025.
+ Each year another 7 million people develop diabetes.
+ Each year 3.8 million deaths are linked directly to diabetes-related causes, including cardiovascular disease made worse by diabetes-related lipid disorders (high cholesterol) and hypertension.
+ Every 10 seconds a person dies from diabetes-related causes.
+ Every 10 seconds two people develop diabetes.

- In many Asian, Middle Eastern, Caribbean countries, and Oceania, diabetes affects 12–20% of the population.
- Seven out of 10 countries with the highest number of people living with diabetes are in the developing world.
- In 2025, 80% of all diabetes cases will be in low and middle-income countries.
- Just under half of all people with diabetes are between 40 and 59 years of age. More than 70% of them live in developing countries.
- India has the largest diabetes population in the world, estimated at 41 million people (6% of the adult population).
- 4.3% of the population in China is affected by diabetes with the number predicted to exceed 50 million people in the next 20 years.
- Type 1 diabetes, which predominately affects youth, is rising alarmingly worldwide (3% per year).
- Some 70,000 children aged 14 and under develop Type 1 diabetes annually.
- An increasing number of children are developing Type 2 diabetes, in both developed and developing nations.
- Type 2 diabetes has been reported in children as young as eight!
- Reports reveal the existence of Type 2 diabetes in juvenile populations previously thought not to be at risk.

The Economic Effect of Diabetes

In the poorest countries, most of the economic impact from diabetes falls on the shoulders of the diabetic patient and their families. The poorest people afflicted by diabetes in India spend an average of 25% of their income on private care. In the Caribbean and Latin America, diabetics shoulder between 40 and 60% of the cost from their own pockets.[13] The cost of diabetes treatment is growing faster than the global population.[14] According to the International Diabetes Federation:

+ The United States spent approximately 232 billion dollars on diabetes treatment in 2007.
+ By 2025, it is estimated the U.S. will spend more than 302.5 billion dollars per year on diabetes treatment.
+ In industrialized countries, about 25% of the medical expenditures for diabetes go to treating elevated blood sugar; 25% goes to treating long-term complications, largely cardiovascular disease; and 50% is consumed by the additional general medical care that accompanies diabetes.
+ For example, expenditures for a person with diabetes who has end-stage kidney disease are 3–4 times higher than expenditures for a person with diabetes and no complications.
+ In the U.S., acute hospitalizations consume 44% of diabetes-attributable costs; followed by 22% for

outpatient care, 19% for drugs and supplies, and 15% for nursing care.

+ In Latin America and the Caribbean, drugs to reduce blood sugar levels are believed to account for about 50% of all healthcare spending.

Medical Care Spending Disparities (according to the International Diabetes Foundation):

+ More than 80% of expenditures for medical care for diabetes are made in the world's economically richest countries.
+ Less than 20% of expenditures are made in the middle and low-income countries where 80% of the people with diabetes will soon live.
+ The U.S. is home to about 8% of the world's population living with diabetes and spends MORE than 50% of all global expenditures for diabetes care.
+ Europe accounts for another 25% of diabetes care spending.
+ The remaining industrialized countries, such as Australia and Japan, account for most of the rest.
+ In the world's poorest countries, not enough is spent to provide even the least expensive lifesaving diabetes drugs.
+ If nothing changes, this disparity will only increase.

Pancreatic abuse has global ramifications, as you can see.

Even though I believe that diabetes is the "Mother Lode" of chronic illness, I also believe undiagnosed pre-diabetes (obesity, insulin resistance, polycystic ovarian syndrome, metabolic syndrome, etc.) contributes to chronic illness before full-blown diabetes is diagnosed.[15]

So which came first? The chicken or the egg? Did obesity, heart disease, insulin resistance, or diabetes come first? Or did pancreatic abuse come first? My hypothesis is the latter.

CHAPTER SIX

How to Stop the Abuse

"I generally avoid temptation unless I can't resist it."
—*Mae West*

Give Your Pancreas a Break

THE SOLUTION IS SIMPLE: reduce the workload of your pancreas. How is this done? By eating foods that keep your blood glucose between 70 and 100, reducing the consumption of fatty foods that increase your cholesterol, practicing portion control, and EXERCISING!

By monitoring your blood glucose, you will discover what foods create a healthy workload for your pancreas. Keeping a steady metabolic situation will prevent your glucose from spiking and then falling, thus reducing cravings and binge eating. You will see improvements in your energy level, your cholesterol level, sleep patterns, skin, and weight.

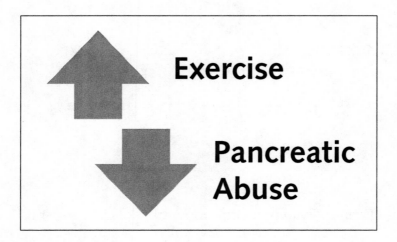

I hear all too often from both morbidly obese and borderline clinically overweight clients—"Eating healthy is so complicated," "It's too expensive," "I am too busy and my life is too crazy to eat this way." Excuses are counterproductive and fall on an unsympathetic ear with me.

Each one of us should strive every day for excellence in everything we do, instead of settling for mediocrity. We are all on this earth for a short time. That time should be filled with a healthy, active lifestyle shared with family and friends, not with doctor's appointments and prescriptions. By taking The Pancreatic Oath and following the PNP guidelines, you are taking the first steps to revolutionize your health and life.

The Pancreatic Nutritional Program (PNP)—
Basic Rules

+ Purchase a glucometer, a scale, and a full-length mirror for daily use.
+ Monitor your blood glucose for 8 to 12 weeks, 4–6 times a day depending on eating patterns. (Diabetics—according to your physician's orders)
+ Maintain the PNP Nutrition and Lifestyle Journal
+ Avoid processed foods.
+ Avoid sugars (artificial or regular).
+ Avoid products with high fructose corn syrup.
+ Avoid dairy (yogurt, cheese, milk, butter, ice cream).*
+ Practice proper food combinations.
+ Take vitamins with physician approval.
+ Avoid soda—that includes all diet drinks.
+ Drink more water.
+ Eat more plant-based protein (beans, tofu, tempeh, etc.).
+ Eat more green leafy vegetables.
+ Eat more whole grains.
+ Eat fruit separately (variety and portion—based upon your reaction to it).

---

*Children and pregnant women need calcium. The restriction of dairy should be an issue between the patient and their physician. Calcium rich foods (kale, for example) and/or supplements may be suggested with the avoidance of dairy.

+ Avoid or limit animal protein. No meat, or if you must—please limit your meat consumption to grass fed, humanely raised beef, pork, lamb, or free-range chicken and turkey that are hormone and antibiotic free.*
+ Limit salt intake.
+ Focus on unprocessed carbohydrates.
+ Stay away from fruit juice (it is high in sugar).
+ No white—white flour, bread, rice, potatoes, pasta.
+ No dried fruits.
+ No smoking.
+ Limit or eliminate alcohol consumption.

You are aware of the connection between mind, body, and spirit. You don't have to read a litany of self-help books to know this intrinsic connection. Your spirit resides in a precious vessel, your body. Your body is sacred and it should be cherished and respected—never abuse it. It is your mind that must make proper choices that either honor the body and spirit or destroy them.

Remember, most chronic illnesses in the U.S. are man-made illnesses. The diet and lifestyle changes advocated by *The Pancreatic Oath* are changes that my family, clients, and I made and continue to thrive as a result. Following the PNP is our way of life. The positive results are definitely worth the small effort this program takes.

---

*Cows were never supposed to graze on corn! Neither were fish. Many farm-raised fish are being fed corn, too! This "fattens" the cow or fish and when you eat it, it will fatten YOU! For more on this, read *The Omnivore's Dilemma* by Michael Pollan.

Do Not Fear the D Word

Somewhere along the way, the word "diet" became a four-letter word. In its purest sense, a diet is simply a course by which people eat. Diets can be strict, such as those imposed in the hospital before and after surgery. Diets often become fads, acquiring a huge following only to fall out of favor in a few years. In any case, in Western societies the word "diet" has become synonymous with the concept of weight loss, even though some diets are aimed at weight gain (for example, the medically prescribed diet for underweight newborn babies). However, since the word "diet" has been inextricably linked to weight loss in our shared culture, I am choosing not to use that word. While people will lose weight if they subscribe to the Pancreatic Nutritional Program™ (PNP), that is not its main purpose.

Honor your body! Say NO to processed foods, sugars, old eating habits and YES to your pancreas!

Instead of a "diet," the PNP is a transformative, healthy eating lifestyle with guidelines that will enable you to figure out what foods are bad for your pancreas and what foods are good for your pancreas. By helping your pancreas, your body will benefit as the weight melts from your frame. The other reason I do not call the PNP a diet is that the plan is individualized for each patient. A typical diet book usually prescribes a "one size fits all" approach with everyone advised the same "induction" and "maintenance" steps.

The PNP does not involve a universal mandate on what you should eat, nor does it contain complicated phases that offer initial water weight loss and eventual gain once the reader attempts to enter the "maintenance" phase.

On the PNP, your body tells you what you can and cannot eat. By checking the glucometer readings of your blood glucose, weighing yourself daily, and checking out your naked body in the mirror on a daily basis as well, you will learn what it needs to eat in order to thrive. I am suggesting that you follow the basic guidelines that will enable you to customize your own eating plan based on your blood glucose.

+ The mirror doesn't lie.
+ The scale doesn't lie.
+ The glucometer doesn't lie.

The first 8–12 weeks of the PNP require self-administered blood glucose level tests taken first thing in the morning in a fasting state and approximately 90 minutes after a meal with the glucometer. The results will provide you with an understanding of how your pancreas processes the foods you eat. Blood glucose is the gauge. *Your task is to keep your blood glucose level between 70 and 100.* These numbers reflect what I and many endocrinologists consider to be an acceptable range. Under 70 is too low and in the hypoglycemic range. Regularly above 100 after certain meals reveals that this food combination does not work for your body. Recipes, food choices and food combinations must be tweaked to yield a post-meal test within the 70–100 range, or the dish must be eliminated from your diet if it continues to spike your blood sugar to an unhealthy range. Through the 8–12 weeks of testing, you will learn what foods, drinks, and even life stressors have a negative impact on your pancreas. You will be able to create the optimal diet for you. The PNP is actually the UN-DIET. It can be adapted to your eating preferences. So, whether you are an omnivore, vegetarian, vegan, or raw foodist, you can use the PNP guidelines to make sure your dietary choices are supporting your health by keeping your blood glucose in a healthy range.

> *The ultimate goal should always be the promotion of pancreatic health by reducing its workload and preventing pancreatic burnout.*

CHAPTER SEVEN

How to Get Started

"Respect your efforts; respect yourself. Self-respect leads to self-discipline. When you have both firmly under your belt, that's real power."
— *Clint Eastwood*

1. Before you begin the PNP, make an appointment with your physician and respectfully **request blood work**. This will provide a point of comparison when you return to your physician in 3 to 6 months after adhering to the PNP. Take the book along. I encourage you to share *The Pancreatic Oath* with your physician. Many of these blood tests are considered routine, but make sure they are included in your blood test results:
   a. Fasting cholesterol, also known as a lipid panel
   b. Fasting glucose
   c. Thyroid function tests

    d. Comprehensive metabolic panel

    e. Liver panel

    f. Adolescent and adult females suffering from symptoms of polycystic ovarian syndrome (PCOS) should request follicle stimulating hormone (FSH), luteinizing hormone (LH) and testosterone levels.

2. At this appointment, **discuss your plan** to improve your health through healthy eating, vitamins, and exercise **with your physician**. Your physician should be your partner and be kept informed about your desire to improve your health. Ask if there are any health issues you might have that would be affected by living the PNP lifestyle and by taking the vitamins suggested in *The Pancreatic Oath.*

3. **Purchase a glucometer.** I do not endorse any particular brand. If you have diabetes, you are presumably already using a glucometer, lancets, and test strips each day. If you do not have a diagnosed condition that requires you to test yourself routinely, you will need to incorporate that habit and expense into your life, but only for a short time. The deal is this: if you test yourself for 8 to 12 weeks, you will have a good understanding of what healthy eating is for you! The meters are not expensive; however, the test strips and the lancets can

> *Be a REBEL! Rebel against advertisers, marketing mavericks, food conglomerates, and anything or anybody who wants to sabotage your health and overwork your pancreas.*

be. The business model for home glucose monitoring is the same as it is for inkjet printers: the printers are cheap or even free, but the specialized ink cartridges are expensive. Money is made not in the purchase of a glucometer, but in the test strips and lancets. In fact, manufacturers often provide free glucometers. Check the internet or ask your pharmacist or physician. If your current glucose is abnormally high, you may get a prescription from your physician and a majority of your expenses may be covered by insurance.

4. **Vitamins.** Take *The Pancreatic Oath* with you to a vitamin store and have the clerk assist you in picking out the vitamins from the list on page 88. **CAUTION:** The vitamins listed are suggestions. They are not endorsed or prescribed. I only share with the reader what has worked for me and for my clients. *Always discuss vitamins with your physician*. Many vitamins can have an adverse effect when mixed with the medication you might be taking already. An example: Vitamin E can interfere with the anti-coagulant medication Coumadin. Also, many vitamins can cause problems if taken in wrong dosages. CoQ10 can also impact the effectiveness of Coumadin.

5. Purchase **a scale** if you do not have one. You should get in the habit of weighing yourself every day. When the weight begins to melt away, it will provide encouragement. If you gain weight, you will know you overdid it the day before. Pancreatic abuse will show up in your blood glucose numbers and on the scale.

6. **Clean out your cabinets and pantry** of any foods that are processed, out of date and contain high fructose corn syrup or trans fats.

7. **Rid your home of soda** (diet or regular). Toss or give away food in your cabinet and refrigerator that have ingredients you cannot pronounce or recognize. Rid your fridge of dairy, sugar-laden **and sugar-free** products. Instead, purchase *unsweetened* products. Healthy eating does not have to be expensive. It is better to eat less of quality products than more of junk. Besides, the investment made in your food is far less than the costs associated with medical care related to a poor diet.

8. When possible, **support your local farmers' market** before going to the grocery store. Making the connection between the sources of your food and your health is crucial to long-term success of the PNP in your life.

9. Take time to experiment with your diet. Try different cuisines, spices, and recipes out. **Cook more. Eat out less.**

10. Stretch, deep breathe, and pamper yourself in small ways daily. Learn to **comfort yourself with things and activities other than food**.

PNP Grocery List

Vegetables:

- Greens: Kale, Swiss Chard, Romaine, Spinach, Cabbage, Collard, Arugula, Dandelion, Endive, Lettuce
- Cucumbers
- Celery
- Leeks
- Onions
- Peppers
- Zucchini
- Broccoli
- Cauliflower
- Bok Choy
- Brussels Sprouts
- Fennel
- Ginger
- Okra
- Sprouts
- Tomatoes
- Mushrooms—Portobello, Shitake, Cremini, Oyster, etc.
- Spaghetti squash
- Butternut squash
- Eggplant
- Artichoke
- Asparagus
- Avocado (though technically a fruit, on the PNP it counts as a fatty vegetable)
- Sweet Potatoes and Yams
- Snow and Sugar Snap Peas
- Radishes
- Garlic
- Fresh herbs—Dill, Basil, Cilantro, Parsley, Mint, etc.

Fruit:

- Apples
- Bananas
- Pears
- Blueberries
- Raspberries
- Grapefruit
- Lemons
- Limes

Deli:

+ Oven-roasted turkey breast (antibiotic and hormone free)
+ Vegan cold cuts and sausages from brands like Field Roast
+ Guacamole
+ Hummus
+ Salsa

Cereals:

+ Oatmeal (extra thick rolled oats, whole grain—**NOT INSTANT**)
+ Uncle Sam Multigrain
+ Granola (low sugar and natural/minimally processed ingredients)
+ Grape-Nuts
+ Quinoa Flakes

Pasta, Rice and Grains:

+ Whole wheat, brown rice, Jerusalem artichoke, quinoa or kamut pasta
+ Shirataki noodles
+ Quinoa
+ Amaranth
+ Brown rice
+ Kasha
+ Barley
+ Bulgur

Breads, Wraps and Crackers:

Look for bread with less than six ingredients—basic bread includes flour, yeast, salt, and water.

Avoid breads with corn flour in the list of ingredients. Look for "gluten-free" products if you have celiac concerns.

Alert—breads, wraps and crackers may increase your glucose. Avoid until achieving weight loss and healthier blood glucose levels. Always limit amount/portion of bread/cracker servings.

+ Rye
+ Pumpernickel
+ Seven Grain
+ Rye, whole grain crackers
+ Natural tortilla chips without salt

+ Wasa crackers
+ Doctor Kracker—Eight Whole Grain Flatbreads
+ Hummlinger Whole Kernel Rye Bread
+ Rice Paper
+ Nori Sheets

Baking:

+ Whole wheat, oat, coconut or gluten-free flour
+ Ener-G Egg Replacer
+ Cacao powder
+ Liquid Stevia
+ Agave
+ Brown rice syrup

+ Maple syrup
+ Blackstrap molasses
+ Raw honey (local)
+ Alcohol free vanilla extract
+ Arrowroot powder

Milks:

+ Unsweetened Almond Milk
+ Unsweetened Coconut Milk
+ Unsweetened Hemp Milk

Refrigerated Case:

+ Organic egg whites
+ Organic free-range eggs
+ Good Belly—a pro-biotic (dairy free) drink
+ Vegan cheese, like rice cheese (Check ingredients to ensure it is "casein free"—which means "dairy free.")
+ Herring
+ Firm tofu
+ Tempeh (fermented tofu)
+ Organic sauerkraut
+ Cream cheese substitute (non-dairy)
+ Sour cream (non-dairy)
+ Earth Balance (Soy-Free Butter Spread) or Ghee
+ Flax oil

Frozen:

+ Non-GMO soy or grain veggie burgers
+ Fish burgers
+ Fish—variety (I prefer buying it fresh; however, if frozen—make sure the fish is wild caught because most farm-raised fish are fed ground corn.)

+ Fish burgers
+ Shrimp, scallops, mussels
+ Frozen vegetables
+ Frozen fruit
+ Edamame
+ Gardein meat substitutes (those products that are low sugar, no sauces)
+ Hemp bagels, bread and other gluten-free breads

Meat Department:

Reduce the amount of animal protein you eat during the week. If you eat meat, use it as a condiment (rather than the main event).

+ Lean, hormone and antibiotic free, sustainably fed, humanely raised meats
+ Wild-caught fish

Seeds and Nuts:

+ Pumpkin seeds
+ Sunflower seeds
+ Poppy seeds
+ Raw almonds
+ Sesame seeds
+ Flax seeds
+ Hemp seeds
+ Chia seeds
+ Walnuts
+ Pecans
+ Pistachio nuts
+ Macadamia nuts (small amounts)
+ Brazil nuts (small amounts)
+ Pine nuts (watch for sensitivity)

Canned and Dry Good Staples:

✦ Beans (If canned—buy organic, in BPA-free cans from brands like Eden Foods and rinse thoroughly.) —lentils, pinto, kidney, black, navy, garbanzo
✦ Organic vegetable broth or organic chicken broth
✦ Organic tomato sauce, diced tomatoes, tomato puree
✦ Organic, meatless, non-creamy pasta sauce (Check labels—avoid sauces with any sugar, including high-fructose corn syrup.)
✦ Raw unsweetened almond butter
✦ Decaffeinated coffee or Yerba Mate (Java Mate is the coffee substitute.)
✦ Vega Protein Powder

Condiments:

✦ Extra virgin olive oil
✦ Unsweetened ketchup
✦ Dijon mustard
✦ Toasted sesame oil
✦ Coconut oil
✦ Apple cider vinegar, Balsamic vinegar (use sparingly), red and white wine vinegars
✦ Vegenaise (instead of mayo; preferred—Grapeseed Oil or Omega-3)
✦ Sea salt

+ Briannas "Real French Vinaigrette"
+ Tamari

Spices:

+ Oregano
+ Bay leaves
+ Cinnamon
+ Cumin
+ Dill
+ Rosemary
+ Cayenne pepper
+ Mustard seeds
+ Nutmeg
+ Paprika
+ Thyme
+ Sage

+ Curry
+ Fennel
+ Chipotle
+ Caraway
+ Turmeric
+ Sage
+ Tarragon
+ Garlic powder
+ Onion powder
+ Black pepper
+ Preservative-free hot sauce

Miscellaneous:

+ Herbal teas—have fun picking out different flavors.
+ Laxative Tea Smooth Move or Super Dieter's Tea [**You may drink one cup at night (before going to bed) ONCE a week if you have trouble with regularity or after you have abused your pancreas by eating a meal laden with junk. Remember, you should not drink it the night before a big meeting or business trip—for obvious reasons!**]

Vitamins

This is a suggested vitamin list. Dosages apply to adults. **Consult with your physician prior to starting with vitamins.**

The Ten PNP™ Essentials

1. Either "RAW" or "ALIVE" brand multivitamins (pick gender specific product)
2. CoQ10—100 mg (Ubiquinol for those over 40 years of age)
3. Stress B-Complex capsules with Vitamin C (should contain 1000 mg of Vitamin C)
4. Vitamin D—2000 IU
5. Cinnamon—1000 mg (recommended for diabetics; however, may increase blood glucose readings)
6. Calcium, Magnesium and Zinc (calcium—1000 mg; magnesium—200–400 mg; zinc—12–15 mg)
7. Fish oil—total Omega-3: 1600 mg (EPA—800 mg; DHA—500 mg)
8. GTF Chromium—200–400 mcg. Taken with meals and/or before workouts (no more than three times per day)
9. Curcumin (Turmeric)—1000 mg
10. Cayenne—450 mg (taken with meals as a metabolism booster)

Take **#1, 2, 3, 4, 8** and **9** in the morning;
OR

Take **#1, 8** and **9** with breakfast and take **#2, 3** and **4** instead of a morning snack with a cup of tea.

Take **#5** IF you are a diabetic with breakfast, lunch and dinner. If it raises your blood glucose, discontinue only AFTER you have ruled out foods that might have triggered a rise in your glucose.

Take **#8** and **9** with breakfast, lunch, and dinner.

Take **#10** with lunch and dinner.

Take **#6** and **7** at bedtime; magnesium promotes sleep.

An easy way to sort this all out is to take snack bags and place the appropriate vitamins in each bag. Label each bag: "breakfast"—"mid-morning snack"—"lunch"—"dinner"—"bedtime."

Candice's Cold/Flu Buster Combo

Garlic capsules
Chewable Vitamin C (1000 mg) tablets

With the first sign of a cold or flu—take a garlic capsule three times a day (morning, noon and night). Chew one Vitamin C tablet three times per day (morning, noon, and night). Drink hot water with lemon throughout the day.

Bowel Stimulator

Super Dieter's Tea or Smooth Moves—use once a week if you have a problem with regularity or after you have stressed your pancreas by eating a pancreatic abusive meal. Remember: never drink either tea the night before a big meeting or day of travel. I think you know why! Also, do not drink Super Dieter's Tea 1–2 weeks before a colonoscopy because the tea can "stain" the lining of your colon.

Why Vitamins?

It is quite simple. Unfortunately, most of the food we eat is nutrient deficient. In the U.S., seeds (many genetically modified) are planted in nutrient poor soil using synthetic fertilizers. As the seeds grow into seedlings/plants, they are sprayed with pesticides. Couple this with fruits and vegetables that are picked too early, shipped long distances, refrigerated, over-cooked—and you have food with questionable nutritional value. In addition, the consumer is leading a stressed, hectic life that affects their food choices—often leading to fast food or processed food high in calories and not nutrient dense. Before you know it, there is a need for vitamins.

My list of suggested vitamins and supplements is short—only ten. A couple of the vitamins have greater value in therapeutic dosages and ONLY under the supervision of a physician or healthcare provider. Don't attempt to increase the amount and play doctor. Leave it to the professional.

Why a Multivitamin?

Multivitamins contain the basic vitamins and minerals. They serve as a safeguard, especially for those who do not eat the recommended servings of fruits, vegetables, etc.

Why CoQ10?

CoQ10 has been associated with slowing the aging process. It helps cells produce energy, especially in the "electrical systems" of the brain, heart, and nerves. CoQ10 is an antioxidant—protecting heart tissue, enhancing the immune system, and even working to fight cancer. CoQ10 is a cell growth regulator. It also protects against diabetes and heart disease (arrhythmias, high blood pressure, and congestive heart failure). It has been used in the treatment of tinnitus (ringing in the ears), senility, Alzheimer's disease, and male infertility (low sperm count). It also reduces fatigue. "Ubiquinol" (suggested for those over 40 years of age) just refers to what "ubiquitous" means: "widespread." It is more thoroughly absorbed.

Coumadin ALERT—CoQ10 could decrease the body's response to Coumadin.

Why Stress B-Complex with Vitamin C?

The following is a breakdown of what makes up B-Complex with Vitamin C.

Why B1 (Thiamine)?

Thiamine enhances brain function, supports metabolism (especially glucose metabolism necessary for a healthy nervous system), can prevent or slow the progression of

Alzheimer's disease, and aids in tissue healing. It has been used to treat disorders of the nervous system like multiple sclerosis, neuritis, and Bell's palsy.

Why B2 (Riboflavin)?

Vitamin B2 is important for the formation and maintenance of eye tissue; aids in treating fatigue and stress, migraine headaches, and skin conditions; may prevent cancer of the bowel.

Why B5 (Pantothenic acid)?

It is called the anti-stress vitamin because it supports the adrenal glands. It works along with Vitamin C to increase cell metabolism of fats and carbohydrates and to promote skin/wound healing.

Why B6 (Pyridoxine)?

Vitamin B6 is needed by the body to turn food into energy and promotes protein metabolism and healthy nerves. It can be used for symptoms of PMS (premenstrual syndrome): nausea, water retention, etc.

Why B12 (Cobalamin)?

Vitamin B12 helps to produce nerve coverings necessary for general growth and appetite, supports red blood cell production, and increases energy. It is especially important for vegans and raw foodists to take B12 as a precautionary measure, since nutritionally it is only found in animal products.

Why Biotin?

Biotin has an important role in producing amino and fatty acids. It is taken with some weight reduction diet programs, used by diabetics to support metabolism, and is important for maintaining healthy skin and hair.

Why Folic Acid?

Folic acid is essential to metabolic function, protein and amino acid metabolism, and red blood cell formation.

Pregnant women need more folic acid as deficiencies are associated with neurological birth defects. Pregnant women must speak with their obstetrician about the proper dosages.

Why Choline?

Choline helps use and move fats between cells, particularly in the liver. It is an important substance in nerves that facilitate nerve transmission for muscle movement and brain function; also used to treat Alzheimer's disease.

Why Vitamin C?

Needed for the production of collagen and cartilage—both necessary for bone growth and bone health. An immune system supporter, Vitamin C protects cell membranes from toxic wastes. It is also an anti-viral agent, an antioxidant, and increases tissue strength.

Why Vitamin D?

Vitamin D is the "sunshine" vitamin. It is necessary for the body to absorb and utilize calcium. Skin produces Vitamin D when exposed to sunlight. So you can imagine if you live in a cold climate, bundled in winter clothing for a good part of the year with little sunshine, how that can affect your Vitamin D levels. You can also understand how it affects the calcium in your bones and teeth. Vitamin D helps the absorption of phosphorous and calcium (important for strong bones), prevents tooth decay, and it also helps bones heal after a fracture.

Why Inositol?

It moves fats from the liver and is important for hair and skin. Therapeutic doses have had a positive effect on Alzheimer's patients—ONLY under the supervision of a physician.

Why PABA (Para-aminobenzoic acid)?

Important in protein metabolism and blood cell formation. Promotes intestinal health and improves hair and skin.

Why Cinnamon for Diabetics?

Dr. Alam Khan of Pakistan and Dr. Richard Anderson of the United States collaborated on a study about 10 years ago to determine whether cinnamon improved blood glucose, triglyceride, total cholesterol, HDL cholesterol, and LDL cholesterol levels in people with Type 2 diabetes.

They found that patients with Type 2 diabetes who took one, three, or six grams of cinnamon per day reduced their serum glucose, triglyceride, LDL cholesterol, and total cholesterol levels—reducing risk factors associated with diabetes and cardiovascular diseases.

Why does cinnamon elevate the glucose levels of some of my clients? I don't have a scientific answer for that. My "guesstimation" is that the percentage of carbohydrates in the cinnamon might cause the spike.

Why Calcium, Magnesium, and Zinc?

Calcium: crucial for bone health; prevents tooth decay; can reduce menstrual cramps and muscle cramping; has been known to promote sleep.

Magnesium: also promotes sleep; important for metabolic function: protein synthesis, neuromuscular function, and energy production; relaxes muscles, even the heart muscle; known to relieve anxiety and stress. It helps with constipation, too.

Zinc: enhances prostate and reproductive health; necessary for adolescents during sexual development; aids in alcohol and amino acid metabolism; protein digestion; extremely important in the body's fight against free radicals; necessary for immune function.

Why Fish Oil?

Regulates inflammation in the body; reduces the thickness and stickiness of blood—keeps it "thin" and moving/

circulating; lowers cholesterol and triglyceride levels; can have a positive effect on arthritis or osteoarthritis, eczema, psoriasis, diabetes, asthma, heart arrhythmias, colitis, and Crohn's disease.

Why GTF (glucose tolerance factor) Chromium?

Improves the body's sensitivity to insulin, thus metabolism is more efficient; may also improve blood lipid profiles such as triglycerides and LDL cholesterol; popular with weight loss programs.

Why Garlic?

It is a natural antibiotic and an antioxidant.

Why Curcumin (Turmeric)?

Increases HDL; lowers LDL; used to prevent and treat Alzheimer's disease and other neurodegenerative disorders; anti-inflammatory; can decrease symptoms of gout and arthritis; can protect the liver; can suppress proliferation of wide variety of tumor cells—some studies suggest it can inhibit cancer metastasis.

Why Cayenne?

Can reduce appetite; increases metabolism; helps rid the body of LDL and triglycerides; it is anti-bacterial; stimulates peristalsis—good for the stomach and intestines; possible anti-cancer agent (lung cancer study at Loma Linda University in California).

Which Would You Rather Spend Your Money On?

Food or medicine?

Truly think about that question.

You will HAVE to open your wallet at some point.

Will it be for good wholesome food or will it be for medicine?

One can be delicious and the other can be literally hard to swallow.

Your choices will cost you—either at the grocery store or the pharmacy. It is your call.

I firmly believe Food is a form of Medicine.

Your body has the ability to heal itself from many conditions if given the proper tools, i.e. healthy choices and amounts of wholesome food grown in an environmentally responsible manner.

CHAPTER EIGHT

The Program

"The first wealth is health.
— *Ralph Waldo Emerson*

I REFER TO *The Pancreatic Oath*'s program as the Pancreatic Nutritional Program (PNP)™. A precious client that I introduced you to earlier, Francine, after three weeks on the PNP, said, "For the first time in my life, I'm in control . . . not food, nor any diet!"

Step 1—Remember Your Goals

You have gone to your physician, had your blood work done, and purchased a glucometer. Great! You are ready to begin. Remember the goals of the program:

✦ Maintain your blood glucose between 70 and 100.

* To place less stress on your pancreas through proper nutrition and exercise.
* To reduce the dosage and number of medications you currently take.
* To live a life filled with good health.

You are NOT on a diet. By taking *The Pancreatic Oath* (page 131), you understand the role you play in your health and your weight. You accept responsibility for yourself and your well-being; and you understand that the PNP is a *lifestyle* for the rest of your life!

The Pancreatic Oath recommends a blood glucose reading between 70 and 100. For those of you that are relatively healthy, it will not take much effort to maintain blood sugars in this range. On the other hand, if you are a Type 2 diabetic, a reading between 70 and 100 may seem virtually impossible. Consider the goals set by your physician. A more realistic range may be between 85 and 180 if you are a diabetic. Do not despair. Instead, reflect on what you ate and what part of the meal might have contributed to your increased numbers. Slowly, but surely on the program, you will move closer to my target optimal range.

As a side note, I want to share an experience with you that was disheartening to me. I attended a Juvenile Diabetes Research Foundation (JDRF) event several months ago. The president of a JDRF chapter and father of a diabetic son addressed the attendees stating he looked forward to the day his son would receive an artificial pancreas so that he could eat anything he wants. RED FLAG! No one should eat anything they want to eat. Thinking like that is precisely why the population is in the state it's in. The end goal of diabetes treatment should not be for everyone to enjoy candy bars and fast food without consequence.

Remember—although the goal is 70–100, it will take time. Diabetics may never achieve those numbers; however, the closer you get, and the less demand you have for insulin, the better it is for your body and your future health. For those who have abused their pancreas and their body for a long time, it will take *time* to heal your body. Even so, you should see a difference in as little as four weeks.

WARNING: Never allow your blood sugar to drop below 70. It can cause you to feel lightheaded, anxious, shaky, and can induce cravings. If you fall too low, you will become ravenous and grab anything and stuff it in your mouth. This will raise your blood sugar, thus raising your insulin level (pancreatic abuse), and propel you into a spiraling situation—eating the wrong foods overly raises your blood glucose, and in turn raises your insulin, which causes your blood glucose to drop, and then again you consume the wrong food and/or drink. This vicious cycle impedes your health and your weight loss.

Special Group—People with Diabetes

Diabetics (Type 1 and 2) MUST remember that as your glucose numbers come down, you MUST adjust your medications (whether oral or injectable insulin). Insulin-dependent diabetics may need to test before they eat as well. Always consult your physician. Your physician will be pleased to partner with you in your quest for improved health. **Exercise and diabetes:** If you are a diabetic and engage in vigorous exercise, remember to test your blood glucose BEFORE and AFTER exercising. Your medication/insulin needs will significantly change due to healthier eating combined with increased exercise/activity. Never allow your blood glucose to dip below 70 or 65. Diabetics must remember to carefully monitor their blood glucose. As they eat "pancreatic friendly" foods, their medication needs (oral hypoglycemic and insulin) will decrease. They must test and be vigilant about dosages to prevent hypoglycemic episodes. In addition, anyone on blood pressure medication should be in contact with their physician before and during the first three months on the PNP. Living the PNP lifestyle will have an effect on their blood pressure, and a reduction in blood pressure medication may be necessary. Your physician is your partner in health. Communication is key.

> *Cardiovascular disease occurs two to four times more in diabetic patients.*

Special Group—People with Cancer

Any person diagnosed with cancer or going through cancer treatments should closely watch their glucose levels and the amount of animal protein consumed. Though this may be controversial, it has a solid rationale. Cancer cells thrive in glucose—they divide and multiply more rapidly. Insulin also affects cancer cells. Andrew Flood, Ph.D., assistant professor in the Division of Epidemiology and Community Health at the University of Minnesota School of Public Health and the University of Minnesota Cancer Center, states, "In general, the idea is that if elevated insulin levels create a biochemical environment conducive to cancer growth, it provides one mechanism by which diet and lifestyle can really influence cancer risk." For this reason, cancer patients should not provide cancer cells with a fertile breeding environment. Please read Dr. T. Colin Campbell's book, *The China Study,* and discuss it with your oncologist. The role of glucose, insulin, and the consumption of animal protein in cancer metabolism remains an important area of future cancer research.

You should be in a partnership with your physician. I cannot stress this enough. It is not, nor should it ever be, a one-sided responsibility. Your health care professional and your body will benefit from **YOUR** participation in **YOUR** health care. You have a responsibility. Do what you can so that medical treatment is more effective. A healthier, nutritionally sound body will be in a better state to withstand the demands of a treatment, be it chemotherapy and/or radiation.

Step 2—Test Your Blood Glucose Level

By now, you should understand that a fundamental component of this program is to test the level of glucose in your blood. Yes, this means using a needle to lance your skin and obtain a drop of blood. If you have diabetes, you are an old pro at this. If you do not have diabetes yet, it may take some time getting used to this.

There will likely be instructions included with your blood glucose meter. Follow them as closely as you can. While meters will have subtle differences in how they function, the basics are the same. First, make sure your hands are clean. This means not only washing your hands thoroughly, but also cleaning the area that you are going to prick with an alcohol swab. The alcohol kills the germs that are on the surface of the skin.

The nerves of the finger course down through the palm side and bend around the tip to the nail and then the nail bed. This means that there are fewer nerves on the sides of the fingers. This is where you should obtain blood as painlessly as possible. When sticking yourself, remember to alternate fingers. For example, prick the little finger of your left hand to test upon rising—then prick the little finger on your right hand 90 minutes after breakfast, followed by the left ring finger and so on.

Blood glucose meters (glucometers) differ in some aspects of information storage and sample size needed, but generally they are the same in function. You will place a test strip in the machine (glucometer), prick your finger, and then place a drop of blood on a test strip. The meter will automatically sense the amount of glucose in your blood and give you a digital reading.

Before you begin the PNP, eat the way you would normally eat for two to five days. Test first thing in the morning for your fasting blood glucose and 90 minutes after you finish eating your meals. This will provide a base line and illustrate the abuse you have been inflicting upon your pancreas. It will establish where you are and show you, later on, how far you have come.

Adjustment Phenomenon

Important to note that initially some non-diabetic clients who have abused their pancreas for many years may test within the normal range—70–100 even though they are eating an unhealthy diet (their pancreas is working very hard). However, their body's voice is heard in their "barrel-like middle" in the abdominal section, increased weight, and unhealthy blood work (cholesterol, triglycerides, creatinine, etc.). **Interestingly, after two to three days on the PNP and eating consistently pancreatic friendly foods, their blood glucose numbers begin to register over 100.** This usually lasts for several days. Many clients worry, but it is the body adjusting to a healthier way of eating. After the first week, their blood glucose levels should begin to represent a realistic picture and give "voice" to the body and the pancreas of what foods it can handle and what it cannot handle. You will find out when you test 90 minutes after finishing your meals and snacks.

Step 3—Record the Numbers

Be vigilant about journaling. Refer to Chapter 9—"The Journal." You must write down your glucose reading, what you ate, and what activity you engaged in (whether yoga, spinning, walking, tennis, yard work, or housework). Keep a small notebook in your pocket or purse. It does not need to be fancy—use it to track what you ate, drank, and your blood glucose results, so that you can enter it in your journal at the end of the day. Some clients love using our companion paperback PNP Nutrition Journal, and other more tech savvy clients utilize our online HIPAA compliant journal at www.ILOVEMYPANCREAS.com to track their food, fitness, and blood glucose testing. Do what is most convenient and consistent for you.

Also, keep index cards in a file box. Record meals or snack results in a good glucose reading, write down what you ate and what your number was. Do the same with a disastrous meal (blood glucose levels well above 120; perhaps 160 to 180 with Type 1 and Type 2 diabetics), it needs to be notated as something you shouldn't be eating. Then you can go to your box and see what worked for your pancreas. It takes the stress out of dietary decision making after a hectic day.

Your body has the ability to heal itself—this does not mean you should not seek medical treatment—it means that you have a responsibility and accountability to yourself and your well-being. It is not the responsibility of your health care providers to work magic by undoing years of body abuse. A prescription many times masks the underlying problem. It takes care of the "surface" problem. It is up to you to deal with the "real." Quit looking for quick fixes—gastric bypass, etc.

PNP Guidelines

Guidelines are very simple:

1. No calorie or carbohydrate counting.
2. No strenuous exercising. Many of my clients are unable to exercise—yet they lose 2–3 pounds per week along with improved blood work.
3. Eat at five-hour intervals. Example: breakfast at 7:30 a.m.; lunch at 12:30 p.m.; dinner at 5:30 p.m. In the beginning, you may need snacks because your body and your pancreas will be adjusting to your new eating habits.
4. Test your blood 4–6 times per day (depending on how many meals or snacks you have per day) for eight to twelve weeks (until you understand how your body reacts to what you put in your mouth). Example: test 90 minutes after you finish eating breakfast, snack,

lunch, snack, and dinner. Finished breakfast at 8, test at 9:30; finished snack at 10:30, test at 12; finished lunch at 1, test at 2:30; snack at 3, test at 4:30; dinner at 6, test at 7:30. You may test up to two hours after eating; however, do not test after two hours because the result will not convey the information you need to hear from your body.

5. NEVER eat fruit with anything else. ALWAYS eat fruit alone. (With two exceptions: ½ an apple with unsweetened almond butter, and Candice's Super Smoothie. It may or may not affect your glucose; however, you must check and assess how *YOUR* body reacts.) If you eat a banana in the morning, you must wait 1½ hours before you eat anything else. Conversely, if you had a salad for lunch, you cannot have any fruit until 1½ hours after consuming the salad. Example—if you finished breakfast at 8 a.m., you cannot have fruit for a snack until 9:30 a.m. (and only after you have tested your blood glucose 90 minutes post-breakfast). Also, if you eat that piece of fruit at 9:30 a.m.—you cannot eat anything until 11 a.m. (except for liquids: water, unsweetened ice tea, hot tea, coffee).

6. Omit dairy—until you get your numbers in the healthy zone. Then, only use dairy sparingly (and only use ORGANIC). It is important to do our part to reduce animal abuse and factory farming that leads to global warming.

7. NO SUGAR. NO ARTIFICIAL SUGAR. That means no diet drinks, diet cookies, or ice cream. Once you get

your pancreas in "idle mode," you will not even crave it. If you do—ask yourself if it is worth abusing your pancreas and compromising your health?

> *Artificial sweeteners are just that "artificial" and "sweet"—you don't need it. That's right— NO DIET DRINKS!*

8. Limit or eliminate alcohol for the first eight weeks. Remember, alcoholic beverages can raise your blood sugar. If you have a glass of wine, please have a full glass of water or unsweetened iced tea before you have a second glass of wine.
9. Practice proper food combining.
10. Exercise. Mix it up! Walk; swim; bike; enroll in a yoga or Pilates class—even housework has healthy benefits.
11. Meditate. It is a vacation from worry and so easy! It does not cost anything—you can do it while taking a bath or even riding the bus or train to work.
12. Take vitamins—Please discuss vitamins with your physician. This is critical if you are on prescription medication. Some vitamins can affect medication you have been prescribed. For example, you would not want to take Vitamin E when you are on anti-coagulant therapy (blood thinners such as Coumadin). DO NOT EXCEED recommended doses. Higher doses will not speed weight loss or improve pancreatic function.

Vitamin supplements—The doses are based on the needs and Recommended Daily Allowance of the average adult. Remember, it is always best to receive vitamins through organic food sources; but it is difficult in today's world, so supplementation may be necessary. The vitamins that I have recommended are in addition to a healthy diet.

+ One multivitamin—Raw or Alive Multi-vitamin (pick gender-specific)
+ B-Complex with Vitamin C
+ Cinnamon capsule (1000 mg) if diabetic—with breakfast and dinner (some clients have reported a higher glucose reading after taking it). Discontinue if it does increase your reading.
+ Vitamin D 2000 IU twice a day
+ Magnesium 200–400 mg (Consider a Magnesium and Calcium combination.)
+ Calcium 800–1,200 mg (Again, consider the Magnesium and Calcium combination.)
+ Coenzyme Q10 (if you have cardiac issues, CoQ10 has been noted to promote heart health) 100 mg (Ubiquinol for those over 40 years of age. Warning: speak with your physician—CoQ10 can decrease your response to Coumadin.
+ Garlic capsules (garlic is associated with the prevention of cancer and heart disease) one per day—unless you feel a cold or flu coming on, then take one in the morning, one at mid-day and one in the evening.
+ Fish oil—I prefer the liquid, 1–2 teaspoons a day. Make sure that the Omega-3 Fatty Acids (total

1600 mg) include high levels of EPA and DHA (EPA—800mg and DHA).

+ GTF Chromium (400 mcg) taken at breakfast and dinner OR before a workout
+ Curcumin (1000 mg) for inflammation
+ Cayenne (450 mg) taken with meals to improve metabolism

Food sources of vitamins—Natural vitamin source should be based on PNP guidelines.

+ Mixed carotenoids—pumpkin, sweet potatoes, carrots, butternut squash, tuna, cantaloupe, mangoes, broccoli, apricots, and watermelon;
+ Vitamin A—cod liver oil, egg yolks, butter, raw whole milk, liver;
+ Folic acid—legumes, poultry, tuna, wheat germ, mushrooms, oranges, asparagus, broccoli, strawberries, cantaloupes, bananas, spinach;
+ Vitamin B6—fish, avocados, lima beans, soybeans, chicken, bananas, cauliflower, green peppers, potatoes, raisins, spinach;
+ Vitamin B1—pork, wheat germ, pasta, peanuts, legumes, watermelon, brown rice, oranges, oatmeal, eggs;
+ Vitamin B2—milk, cottage cheese, avocados, tangerines, prunes, asparagus, broccoli, beef, salmon, turkey, mushrooms;

- Vitamin B3—meats, poultry, fish, peanut butter, legumes, soybeans, whole grains, broccoli, baked potatoes, asparagus;
- Vitamin B12—salmon, eggs, cheese, swordfish, tuna, clams, mussels, oysters;
- Pantothenic acid—fish, whole grain, mushrooms, avocados, broccoli, peanuts, cashews, lentils, soybeans, eggs;
- Biotin—oatmeal, nuts, eggs, wheat germ, poultry, cauliflower, legumes;
- Vitamin C—citrus fruit, strawberries, tomatoes, bell peppers, spinach, cabbage, melons, broccoli, raspberries, kiwi fruit;
- Vitamin D—sunlight, butter, tuna, milk, eggs, salmon;
- Vitamin E—nut and vegetable oils, wheat germ, mangoes, blackberries, broccoli, apples, spinach, whole wheat, peanuts;
- Vitamin K—tomatoes, eggs, dairy products, carrots, avocados, spinach, broccoli, cabbage, Brussels sprouts, parsley;
- Calcium—kale, turnip greens, almonds, green beans, milk, cheese, yogurt, salmon, sardines with bones, broccoli, green beans;
- Magnesium—molasses, spinach, wheat germ, nuts, pumpkin seeds, seafood, baked potatoes, broccoli, bananas;
- Selenium—meats, whole grain, dairy products, fish, shellfish, mushrooms, Brazil nuts;

+ Potassium—potatoes, avocados, bananas, yogurt, cantaloupe, milk, mushrooms, tomatoes, spinach.
+ Sodium is also important; however, you get more than enough with your regular diet.
+ Zinc—lean beef, seafood, lima beans, legumes, nuts, poultry, and dairy products.

Pick and choose from the list of natural vitamin sources that follow the PNP guidelines.

CHAPTER NINE

A Day in the Life with *The Pancreatic Oath*'s PNP

PNP Goal—Maintain Blood Glucose **between 70 and 100**.

Eat Main Meals at 5-hour intervals. Example: breakfast at 8:00 a.m.; lunch at 1:00 p.m.; dinner at 6:00 p.m. Mid-morning snack between 10:00 and 11:00 a.m.; mid-afternoon snack between 3:00 and 4:00 p.m. This timeframe is based on a 30-minute meal (finishing breakfast by 8:30 a.m. and then testing at 10:00 a.m. would allow you to snack after testing).

1. **First thing in the morning**
   a. After you awake, sit on the side of your bed and take in three cleansing breaths—inhale, slowing counting 1, 2, 3 and 4; exhale counting backward 4, 3, 2 and 1.

    b. Go to the bathroom. Wash your hands with soap and water.

    c. Check your blood glucose and journal it.

    d. Weigh yourself and journal it.

    e. Freshen up and then pour yourself a cup of hot water. Add a squeeze of fresh lemon juice. You may want more than one cup. This should get your digestive system up and running and stimulate your bowels.

2. **Breakfast**

    a. Eat

        i. plain oatmeal and unsweetened almond milk
   or

        ii. one piece of fruit or a bowl of fruit
   or

        iii. choose from the breakfast list

    b. Beverages

        i. Decaf coffee, green tea, herbal tea, or filtered water

    c. Put a snack bag together of either almonds (no more than 10 per serving) or veggies. Check snack list for other recommendations.

    d. Journal what you ate for breakfast and the time (set alarm for 90 minutes).

    e. Take your vitamins/supplements.

    f. Pack your glucometer.

    g. 90 minutes AFTER eating breakfast, test your glucose and record the results. You may want to set the alarm mode on your cell phone to remind you. Was it high? If so, what choices did you make that you think affected the number?

3. **Snack** (only if you must; between breakfast and lunch, and lunch and dinner).

   Example: if you finished eating at 8:00 a.m. and tested at 9:30, then you could have a snack at 10 or 11. Remember, you have to test 90 minutes after the snack (if you ate a snack at 10:00, then you would test at 11:30).

   I divide my morning vitamins—taking half with breakfast and the other half as my snack with a cup of herbal tea. **Refer to snack list.**

   If you don't snack—you don't have to test.

   a. Journal what you ate and drank for snack (remember to record the time and set alarm for 90 minutes).
   b. Take and journal your blood glucose 90 minutes after finishing your snack.

4. **Lunch**
   a. Mixed salad with salmon (no cheese or bacon)—oil and vinegar dressing
      or
   b. Soup (not milk or cream based; no pasta) and a small house salad—oil and vinegar dressing
      or
   c. Choose from lunch recommendations.
   d. Take mid-day vitamins.

    e. Journal what you ate and drank (remember to record the time and set alarm for 90 minutes later).

    f. 90 minutes later, take and record blood glucose.

5. **Exercise**

    Swim, walk, take a tennis lesson, enroll in a yoga or Pilates class, bike, lift weights, even do housework. Breathe deeply. Don't forget to stretch before or after engaging in any form of exercise.

6. **Dinner**

    a. whole wheat, brown rice, or kamut/quinoa blend of pasta with marinara or any veggie sauce
       or

    b. chicken, turkey, fish, tofu, or tempeh (fermented tofu) with veggies (asparagus or zucchini) and a salad
       or

    c. Refer to dinner recommendations.

    d. 90 minutes later, take and record blood glucose.

    e. Journal what you ate and drank along with the time (set alarm for 90 minutes).

    f. Record blood glucose.

7. **Bedtime**

    a. Before going to bed, have a cup of relaxation tea and take the remainder of your vitamins.

    b. Look over your journal before going to bed. Did your blood glucose soar after any particular meal or snack? What do you think triggered it? Was it the slice of bread you ate? Was it the diet soda you decided to drink? Was it the catsup you added to your sandwich? Was it stress? Did you adhere to proper food combinations?

c. If you have issues with middle-of-the-night eating or you are a diabetic that experiences "high rise" or "Dawn Phenomenon," an elevated fasting blood glucose reading in the mornings—you may have hummus or raw unsweetened almond butter on a couple of celery sticks as a nighttime snack before bed to combat these issues.

Remember:

1. Carbs/starch (a pasta or grain like quinoa) + salad + veggies = **GOOD**
2. Protein (plant based: soy or beans; animal: poultry, fish) + salad + veggies = **GOOD**
3. Soup (not milk or cream based; without pasta) + salad + veggie = **GOOD**
4. Soup (chicken soup) + entrée (carb or protein—pasta or animal protein) + salad = **BAD**
5. Carb (rice, pasta, potatoes) + animal protein (chicken, fish, beef) + salad = **BAD**

"As I see it, every day you do one of two things: build health or produce disease in yourself."
—*Adelle Davis*

> *Remember to test 90 minutes after you eat*
> *(breakfast, snacks, lunch, and dinner)*

Additional Tips:

✦ Avoid or limit alcohol in the beginning. If you do have an alcoholic beverage, limit your intake to two drinks. Remember to have a full glass of water or unsweetened ice tea in between drinks one and two.

✦ Avoid simple refined carbohydrates (snack food, white bread, etc.).

✦ If you are on the run and need to eat at a fast food restaurant:

—You can have a burger (if you must) or grilled fish sandwich (no ketchup—because it has sugar or high fructose corn syrup) with one slice of bun; use lettuce for the top bun. Or, if you eat at a Panera Bread, for example, have a bowl of black bean soup and a small house salad with oil and vinegar.

—Instead of soda, have water or iced unsweetened tea.

—Substitute veggies for potatoes when eating out.

—Never clean your plate—always leave something on it.

> —Substitute salad for toast/muffin/hash browns
> when ordering an omelet.
> —If you have to take a deep breath before your
> next bite—you are FULL—STOP eating!

◆ Eating a simple carbohydrate, starch or sugar, causes an immediate rise in your blood glucose and gives you a surge of energy, but does not contain any valuable nutrients (such as fiber or minerals) to slow down the entry into your system. This causes a quick "high" and a rapid descent "low." Your body is only satisfied for a short time—instead of being satisfied for several hours. You become hungry sooner than later. This becomes a vicious cycle. Eat the wrong food, get hungry one hour later, and then eat the wrong food again. It is pancreatic abuse and promotes poor health.

Be good to your pancreas and
it will be good to you!

Notes on the Glycemic Index

Often clients come to me with questions about the Glycemic Index and how it relates to the PNP.

Applauding the painstaking research that went into creating the glycemic index, I must however address the misconception that all low GI numbers are good or healthy for you. An example: the GI for tomato soup is 39 and the GI for black bean soup is 64. I cannot eat tomato soup—it causes my blood sugar to soar; however, black bean soup keeps my blood glucose under 100. Apple juice has a GI of 40; my pancreas and my body don't see it that way. I can't drink it, because it will spike my glucose.

Old-fashioned oatmeal (made with water) has a GI of 49. Many of my clients can't handle it. Their body/pancreas reacts to it in a negative way by spiking their blood glucose as if they had just eaten one of those sugary cereals marketed to children.

This brings us back to the core of "one size does not fit all." Your body/pancreas will speak to you—it will provide you with an answer 90 minutes after you eat. The number will elicit from the body either a thumbs up or a thumbs down—a "thank you" or "what are you trying to do? I can't work with this, so I guess I'll just *store* it" response. Following the glycemic index is not the same as following the PNP. You still must use the provided protocol to determine categorically if low glycemic foods actually have a low glycemic impact on YOUR blood glucose.

Message about Exercise

The whole notion of "working out to eat" baffles me. Why would anyone jog for miles so that they could eat a hot fudge sundae? You may rid your body of the caloric intake; however, you still have created a toxic environment for your body. By raising your blood glucose to address the hot fudge sundae, you forced the poor pancreas to "rescue" the situation by producing and pumping out enough insulin to stabilize the blood sugar. Doesn't make sense, does it? Exercise won't undo this damage.

Many of my clients are referred because they have tried everything else to improve their health and their physicians don't know what more to do for them. They are compromised, unable to walk or workout due to knee and hip problems, heart disease, obesity, or diabetes. Yet once they begin the PNP, they lose weight, lower their cholesterol, lower their blood pressure, and reduce their need for insulin or oral hypoglycemic agents (Metformin, Glucotrol). They feel better. Think clearer. Move more easily.

That said, I do not recommend vigorous exercise for any of my clients, especially my severely overweight patients. Vigorous exercise can lead to a decrease in blood glucose that can cause an increase in appetite. Moderate exercise is encouraged; however, no amount of exercise will reverse the effects of a poor diet.

In the beginning, walking is best (if they can). As my clients lose weight, reduce or eliminate all medication, they feel better and can physically accomplish more in the area of exercise. They can lose between two and three pounds a week without exercising. Isn't the human body amazing? Just give it the proper tools, i.e. wholesome, nutritious, responsibly grown food, and it does all the work!

By stretching and building functional strength through weight lifting as they progress, they increase their mobility and overall self-sufficiency.

CHAPTER TEN

The Pancreatic Nutritional Program (PNP) Journal

Why Journal?

1. Journaling is a way to maintain accountability. It keeps you honest.
2. The foundation of the Pancreatic Nutritional Program is discovering the connection between your diet, lifestyle, stress level and their impact on your blood glucose level.
3. You need to record data daily in order for the program to be effective and give you a clear picture of what foods and activities support pancreatic health as well as protect the pancreas, provide weight loss and improve health.

4. Photocopy the provided daily journal page on page 126 in a 90-day supply. Punch holes in the pages and place in a ringed binder for your personal tracking. You may want to purchase the companion book—*The Pancreatic Oath Nutrition and Lifestyle Journal* to track your data.

5. Take your journal everywhere or login to our online journal at www.ILOVEMYPANCREAS.COM to track your progress and ultimately, create the best nutrition and lifestyle management program for yourself.

In the beginning, you may feel like journaling is tedious or a waste of time. Change is rarely easy, but the first step is to commit to a meal-by-meal and day-by-day review of your diet and lifestyle. Your journal should be your place to confide and keep things "real." There is no point in lying about what you ate, how much you exercised or fibbing as to what your blood glucose numbers are in a given day. You will only be serving as a roadblock to your best self.

If you are honest in your journal and you commit to testing and recording your data daily, you will see patterns emerge as to what is pancreatic friendly and what is abusive to your pancreas. Tarot readers often describe psychic card readings as your soul's way of speaking to you. Well, what you record in your journal can be viewed as your body's way of communicating to you. It is a miraculous instrument that can and does survive much mistreatment on our parts. However, if we want to honor our physical existences, we must learn from our bodies. What foods and beverages are positive for our particular body and what foods are negative. What our bodies prefer and do not prefer to consume. With a healthy diet, active lifestyle and investment in stress management and holistic personal care, we are giving our bodies the tools needed to heal and be well. We cannot just rely on our physician to rescue us by prescribing medications that mask symptoms, rather than addressing the root cause—the overconsumption of poor food choices coupled with a sedentary lifestyle. We must do our part to improve the state of our health and should look at ourselves as partners with our healthcare providers. We play a vital role in our own wellbeing. Please join me in practicing SELF-HEALTH.

> *Effective health care depends on self-care; this fact is currently heralded as if it were a discovery.*
> *—Ivan Illich*

The Pancreatic Nutritional Program (PNP)™ Journal Instructions:

Date: Enter the date as well as the day of the week in this section. This will help you to determine patterns in your diet, activity and stress levels.

Morning Blood Glucose: Should be taken first thing in the morning after you wake up in a fasting state (before you have eaten or had anything to drink). Ideally, right after you use the bathroom and wash your hands, you should test your blood glucose.

Weight: Weigh yourself first thing in the morning after using the bathroom and before you have consumed any food or drink. Always weigh yourself completely naked and make sure the scale is in the same spot on a solid surface (no carpeting).

Cup of Hot Water: A mug of warmed water with a squeeze of lemon is beneficial for detoxification and stimulating the bowels.

Meal Chart: Record everything you ate and drank for each meal or snack. Record the time you ate. Approximately, 90 minutes later you will test your blood glucose to see the effects of what you ate and drank on your pancreas. To remind yourself when to test add 90 minutes to when you finished eating a meal or snack and place it in the "Time + 1.5 Hours Column." Note which meals and snacks keep your blood glucose within a healthy range.

Speak and work with your physician. If you are a Type 1 or Type 2 Diabetic your need for insulin or oral hypoglycemic agents will change as you improve your diet and lifestyle and lower your blood glucose. Diabetics should be vigilant about monitoring their lowering blood glucose levels. NEVER allow levels to go below 65. Pancreas-friendly meals keep your blood glucose between: 70–100. Diabetics may range between 80–140. Remember *The ultimate goal for diabetics are numbers closer to 100.*

Stress Level: High stress levels can have an adverse effect on blood glucose levels and your long term health. It is important to monitor patterns of stress and develop management techniques. From the scale of 1–10 (with 10 being the most stressed), choose your overall stress level for the day.

Exercise: Moderate exercise is advocated on the PNP. Record your physical activity for the day. Monitor over time what variety of exercise works best for your body.

Meditation/Deep Breathing: Everyday you should take time to reflect and settle your mind, freeing it from family, work and other distractions. Aim for 10–20 minutes a day. In addition, deep cleansing breathes in the morning, at night or whenever needed are effective in managing stress and connecting you with gratitude for the miraculous functioning of your body.

Vitamins: Vitamins are beneficial support tools to your nutrition program. A list of *recommended* supplements may be found on page 88.

Eight Glasses of Water: Proper hydration is crucial to maintaining overall health and achieving weight loss.

DATE _____

MORNING BLOOD GLUCOSE _____

WEIGHT _____

CUP OF HOT WATER   Yes   No

	Meal	Time	Time + 1.5 hours	Glucose at 1.5 hours
Breakfast				
Snack				
Lunch				
Snack				
Dinner				

STRESS LEVEL _____

Low ⟶ High

| 1 | 2 | 3 | 4 | 5 | 6 | 7 | 8 | 9 | 10 |

EXERCISE   Type _____   Yes   No

MEDITATION/DEEP BREATHING   Yes   No

VITAMIN   Yes   No

EIGHT GLASSES OF WATER   Yes   No

PNP™ Meal Discovery Cards

The first page provides an example of how to fill out the PNP Meal Discovery Cards. Make copies of the second page or purchase index cards to keep in a recipe holder. You will use them to record meals that work (and don't work) for your body.

Pancreas-friendly meals keep your blood glucose between: 70–100. For Diabetics, the goal is 80–140.

A meal that raises your blood glucose over 140 should never be a part of your regular diet.

The cards should serve as quick tools to help you in your meal planning.

MY PNP™ MEAL DISCOVERY CARD

Date ___7/4___ Pancreas Friendly____ NOT_✓_

Breakfast ____ Lunch ____ Dinner _✓_ Snack ____

Meal __Fried chicken, macaroni salad, potato,__
__cole slaw, soda__

_____ Glucose __196__

MY PNP™ MEAL DISCOVERY CARD

Date ___8/10___ Pancreas Friendly_✓_ NOT____

Breakfast ____ Lunch _✓_ Dinner ____ Snack ____

Meal __Romaine and mixed green salad, oil &__
__vinegar dressing with boiled salmon, sparkling__
__water__ Glucose __88__

MY PNP™ MEAL DISCOVERY CARD

Date ___9/20___ Pancreas Friendly_✓_ NOT____

Breakfast _✓_ Lunch ____ Dinner ____ Snack ____

Meal __Tofu scramble with vegetables, green tea__

_____ Glucose __80__

MY PNP™ MEAL DISCOVERY CARD

Date _____ Pancreas Friendly____ NOT____

Breakfast ____ Lunch ____ Dinner ____ Snack ____

Meal _____

_____

_____ Glucose _____

MY PNP™ MEAL DISCOVERY CARD

Date _____ Pancreas Friendly____ NOT____

Breakfast ____ Lunch ____ Dinner ____ Snack ____

Meal _____

_____

_____ Glucose _____

MY PNP™ MEAL DISCOVERY CARD

Date _____ Pancreas Friendly____ NOT____

Breakfast ____ Lunch ____ Dinner ____ Snack ____

Meal _____

_____

_____ Glucose _____

CHAPTER ELEVEN

The Ten Commandments of Health and *The Pancreatic Oath*

"One should eat to live, not live to eat."
— *Cicero*

C HANGE CAN BE SIMPLE, yet it is never easy for most of us. The concepts and approach of the PNP are straightforward, but doing it every day, especially in the beginning, can be difficult. Motivation comes from both the mind and the heart. Knowledge of how your body processes the foods you eat motivates the desire for improved health and weight loss.

Throughout the process of change, we all need words and thoughts to help us stay focused and motivated. *The Pancreatic Oath* and The Ten Commandments of Good

Health should be part of your everyday thought process concerning food. Memorize them and apply them.

The Ten Commandments of Good Health

1. Thou shall protect the pancreas.
2. Thou shall avoid processed foods.
3. Thou shall maintain a healthy glucose level.
4. Thou shall exercise and meditate.
5. Thou shall practice proper food combinations.
6. Thou shall read food labels.
7. Thou shall practice portion control.
8. Thou shall eliminate sugars.
9. Thou shall eat fruit separately.
10. Thou shall love, cherish and protect thy health.

The title of this book is *The Pancreatic Oath* because I believe that the health of the pancreas is the key to good health or bad overall health. I also believe that by protecting the pancreas one can avoid or reverse chronic illness that stems from an abused pancreas. Once you truly understand the vital role your pancreas plays in your overall wellbeing, the PNP will become an important and essential component of your life. So much so that you will be willing to take an oath, *The Pancreatic Oath.*

The Pancreatic Oath

I promise to cherish, protect, respect, and nourish my pancreas and my body.

I will abstain from food, drink, and substances that place a burden or have a destructive effect on my pancreas, my body, my mind and my spirit.

I will take responsibility and do all in my power to improve and maintain my health and to prevent illness. I make this pledge not only for me, but also for those entrusted with my care.

CHAPTER TWELVE

Achieving *Self-Health*: Testimonials and Case Studies

Testimonials

"I followed Candice's diet plan one year ago. I was 45 pounds overweight with high blood pressure, a cholesterol problem and Type 2 diabetes. I took off 35 pounds in the eight-week period and continued with another 20 over the year. At a checkup in April, my cholesterol was way down, I was taken off the blood pressure medication and the Metformin for diabetes.

"The weight has stayed off. The eating pattern becomes a way of life. My sugar levels are rarely above 100.

"I do test every morning. I will also, at this point, eat whatever I want when out or at a party and try to keep it in line the next

day. This diet changed my life. I think it is successful because of the immediate reinforcement of testing . . . You are in charge of what goes in your mouth and you can see the result immediately."

—SALLY P.

"Today is the end of 12 weeks. You told me I would lose between 20 and 31 pounds. I ended up at exactly minus 25 pounds . . . Please sign me up for another 12 weeks . . . I was at a wedding with {name removed} and found out she is on the PNP, too! She looks great."

—AL F.

"Candice Rosen and The Pancreatic Oath *changed my life . . . After doing the PNP for eight weeks I felt 10 years younger . . . I had so much energy and felt wonderful . . . I lost 15 pounds in the eight weeks . . . it is still off, over a year later . . . This is the only way to live . . . I highly recommend it to everyone."*

—GINNA B.

"I followed Candice Rosen's weight loss plan and lost 20 pounds in six weeks! I didn't find it very difficult, just a little discipline, and boy, do those pounds fall off. It becomes a way of eating rather than a diet."

—YALE S.

"I came to the Pancreatic Nutritional Program through a referral. My co-worker who was overweight, depressed, and low energy was now getting skinny and full of pep. Her outlook on life was even improving. I had to know her secret. She said it was the PNP!

140

"However, at first, I didn't think it was something that could help me. I was not only overweight and tired, but I was also suffering from Type 2 diabetes and rheumatoid arthritis. When I began my counseling sessions, I didn't really believe in my own ability to impact my health. I couldn't control my emotional eating. I had no understanding of the biology behind my cravings.

"After losing 46 lbs, getting off my medications . . . and finally putting on a bathing suit this vacation (after 15 years of t-shirts and shorts at the beach), I'm a believer! I am in less pain from my arthritis and have even started a low impact exercise routine. My daughters (13 and 19) have now entered the Family Counseling program and they are improving their health, too, by learning how to eat better. I don't want them to suffer as I have over the years. I don't want them to ever resort to yo-yo dieting. The PNP has given us a new outlook on life. I am forever grateful to Candice!"

—MARIA A.

"I was diagnosed at 24 with polycystic ovarian syndrome (PCOS). My symptoms included irregular periods, embarrassing body hair, acne, and a spare tire around my middle. Working with my endocrinologist, my gynecologist, and the registered dietician at the hospital had not made a dent in my symptoms. After entering the Pancreatic Nutritional Program . . . I became hooked on learning more about my body and how simple changes could have a major impact on my health over time. I am mid-way through the PNP Detox now, and I use the tools provided to tweak my diet in order to manage my condition. Instead of trying to mask my symptoms with different medications, I got to the cause of

them . . . I look hot and, more importantly, I feel hot. Finally losing the freshman 15 that stayed on since college."

—LETESHA J.

"When I first began working with Candice and the Pancreatic Nutritional Program I weighed 260 pounds and stood at 5'9". I had horrible eating habits that included eating out for at least one meal of the day, drinking a sugar-filled espresso drink from Starbucks on a daily basis, as well as an addiction to Diet Coke that consisted of at least three Diet Cokes a day. What I find so wonderful about this program is that once you learn the basics of it you can continue with it on your own. The PNP does not have you eat 'their specific food' nor does it require you to count anything—be it calories or points. With the help and instruction of Candice, I was able to lose 25 pounds in eight weeks. I have continued to lose 10 more pounds bringing my total weight down to 225. What I am most grateful for is learning how to look at food and where it belongs in my life. Prior to working with Candice, this was unfortunately not a top priority. I have learned that food is not my main priority and as a result have a much healthier relationship with food as well as its role in my life."

—ALEX F., AGE 26

"I am a marathon runner and an avid cyclist. Even though I was active and the picture of health, inside I was the opposite. I had alarmingly high cholesterol and triglycerides. I thought I was eating healthy and nourishing by body properly. However, at my annual physical I was told I needed to be on a statin drug.

I was beyond confused. My partner told me about the PNP. I entered the program and it changed my life. No medication. No more caffeine addiction. No more headaches. Best part, I now sleep through the night. Thank you, Candice!"

—Bruce W.

"*When I began my journey on the Pancreatic Nutritional Program, I was in a great deal of pain from a back injury. I had two shoulder surgeries in two years. I was a mess. I had been over 200 pounds for more than 20 years. I stood in front of Candice at 230 pounds After that, I did whatever Candice told me to do. I had tried everything under the sun and never lost more than 30 pounds. On some programs, I had even gained weight.*

"*I knew from that morning my life was going to change. Was I hungry? HELL yes, I was, but I felt great. WHY? Because I began to have feelings again. I was no longer clouded by sugar and overeating. I joined a health club. I not only exercised, but I steamed, relaxed, and learned to be quiet. I did small things every day to reward myself. Good books and music. I took Jazz 101 and loved it.*

"*I told my family to feed themselves. Two grown men . . . I thought they could handle that and they did. It took some time, but they also supported my new way of life. My son even likes some of my dinners and joins in. It hasn't been a year yet and I've lost over 75 pounds. I went from a size 20 to size 8 pants! Working out has reshaped my legs and arms. Also, it helped my overall mental health.*

"What was so different from all the other programs I tried the meter (glucometer). The meter was the MAIN KEY! Numbers don't lie. I followed the guidelines of the PNP. What I found out was I was eating all the wrong things. That is why nothing ever worked for me. What the meter taught me was that only I could tell myself . . . what to eat and when to eat.

"I don't like to stuff food in my mouth first thing in the morning. When I was younger, I was skinny, until I had children. I never ate a meal until lunch. When I was on all those other programs, it was Eat! Eat in the morning! Eat! Eat! Eat! You know what all that eating got me in the morning? It just made me want to eat all day long! Now I enjoy hot coffee, then some tea and maybe ¼ of a pear or some nuts in the morning. I don't need that much to get me going.

"I'm 51 and the older I get, the less I need to eat. I've learned also about working out. I was overworking out with a trainer before the PNP. I needed to listen to my body and myself about workouts just like I was doing with my food. More yoga and pool. Less running and lifting.

"Those of us who have struggled with weight loss . . . we are the best excuse-makers in the world. We are better than addicts, or the most cunning of crack heads. We are junkies! Numbers became my life! No more lies to myself.

"Pictures tell a thousand words. Once I saw the pictures of myself at a school reunion . . . I saw myself as everyone else saw me. I was FAT—HUGE at 5'3" and 230 pounds! I looked like a round ball.

"I no longer feel like a round ball or move like one. My life has changed so much because of the PNP. The meter was the key to the food. Most helpful for me were all my one-on-one sessions with Candice. I would have never been able to do all this on my own without Candice. Yes, it was therapy for me. I needed her more than I needed anyone. Her brown eyes were my lifeline for weeks! I never wanted to miss our sessions. I was getting stronger with every session . . . more confident with every pound lost and every weekly meeting . . . learning more about food and then about myself . . . holding that mirror up every day works for me in more ways than one!

"I looked at myself naked that first night I came home from Candice's office and do so every day, because it was and continues to be the naked truth! Candice maintains: The mirror doesn't lie. The scale doesn't lie. The meter doesn't lie. I stopped lying to myself. I look in the mirror every day, I weigh myself every day and I still test every day. It keeps me honest with myself. I will forever be indebted to Candice and the Pancreatic Nutritional Program for helping me find 'My Keys' so I could start the ride of my life."

−P. HALL

Case Studies

Veronica, age 54

Veronica is a 54-year-old well-educated, self-employed, married mother of three children. She has been overweight for the past eight years.

She came to see me during the winter holiday season with a desire to lose weight, improve her blood work and her health. Veronica knew that embarking on a lifestyle change would be difficult considering the upcoming Christmas holidays and her inability to exercise due to the fissures on the bottom of her feet. However, she was committed to improving her health. She complained of being tired and had trouble sleeping. Veronica is 5'6" tall and weighed 167 pounds. She was under the care of a physician and taking Prednisone at the time of her initial visit, along with Metformin 500 mg. She stated it was to offset her elevated blood glucose levels from the Prednisone. She was also taking Levothyroxine 0.75 mg.

Her blood work showed total cholesterol—235; triglycerides—131; HDL—83; LDL—126. Her Vitamin D was low at 28.8 (normal range 32–100).

Approximately 12 weeks later, Veronica weighed 150 pounds and her blood work improved. Total cholesterol—199; triglycerides—91; HDL—89; LDL—92! Vitamin D was no longer an issue. This improvement was accomplished during the holiday season while on Prednisone (for the fissures) even though she was unable to exercise. With a reduction in night sweats, due to menopause, Veronica's sleep improved along with her energy level. She accomplished all of this while on a steroid drug (which causes water retention).*

Sonia, age 56

Sonia is a 56-year-old married mother of three grown children and grandmother of two. She is 5'5" tall, weighed 204 pounds and carried a "barrel" around her middle. Night sweats, her weight, Type 2 diabetes, and the need for hip replacement surgery were her wake-up call. Her inability to exercise due to her hip was an obstacle. Her goals are to lose weight, reduce or eliminate her medication, and prepare her body for hip surgery. Sonia states she is menopausal and suffers from terrible night sweats. Her medication intake included Zetia 10 mg (1 per day), Meloxicam 7.5 mg (1 tablet two times per day), Metformin 500 mg (twice a day), Niaspan 1000 mg (one at bedtime), Amlodipine 10 mg (one per day), and Crestor 40 mg.

The PNP is now a way of life for Sonia. She lost and has kept off a total of 47 pounds. Not only did she lose weight, but she prepared her body for successful hip replacement surgery. She is off medication, sleeps better, and night sweats have been significantly reduced. Sonia is practicing successful *Self-Health* and enjoying a life filled with family, friends, and golf.

---

*Veronica had to resume taking Prednisone twice during the course of the 12-week PNP induction for her feet fissures.

Kate, age 58

Kate presented with metabolic syndrome, high blood pressure, and high cholesterol. Kate is 5′5″ tall and weighed 200 pounds. Her blood work revealed blood glucose—96; A1c—6.1; total cholesterol—308; HDL—68; triglycerides—264; LDL—187.

Eating to protect her pancreas had a profound effect on her blood work two months later with the added bonus of a 20-pound weight loss. Follow-up blood work showed blood glucose—105; A1c—5.8; cholesterol—270; HDL—81; triglycerides—99; LDL—169.

Connie, age 17

Connie is a Type 1 diabetic and a high school senior. She came to see me with her parents because her weight and insulin needs were skyrocketing. Connie is 5′8″ tall and she weighed 169 pounds. She was diagnosed with Type 1 diabetes at age six. She has an insulin pump. She had a baseline of 17 units and then used 60 plus units of Apidra daily. Her increasing weight and need for more insulin, along with night corrections, was alarming to both Connie and her parents.

Within one month, her weight had dropped to 159, her bedtime corrections were few and far between and her blood glucose hovered around 100 instead of 200. Although her basal rate continues at 17, her additional insulin usage has decreased to 30–35 units per day. Two weeks later, her A1c dropped from 8.7 to 8.5. Her endocrinologist's target A1c is 8.0.

Paul, age 65

Paul is dealing with Type 2 diabetes, eyesight problems, weight issues, knee problems, and blood work that indicates heart and kidney problems. His energy level was low and he weighed 265 pounds when he arrived for his first appointment. He was on 50 units of Lantis a day. Blood work revealed A1c—7.5; fasting glucose—123; cholesterol—149; triglycerides—87; HDL—51; LDL—81. Although those numbers look good, they are low due to the medication he is taking. Masking the underlying issue is NOT addressing the problem. The abuse to the body continues with swings in glucose and insulin. This is expressed in Paul's kidney function lab values: creatinine—1.82 (normal: 0.76–1.27); microalbumin (urine)—3528.3 (normal: 0.0–17.0), and microalbumin/creatinine ratio—1340.5 (normal: 0.0–30.0).

After four weeks on the PNP, Paul lost 17 pounds and was walking a 25-minute mile. His breakfast of a Coke is now a thing of the past. At five weeks, his Lantis was reduced to 38 units a day.

At the conclusion of the 12-week PNP, Paul weighed 242 pounds (a loss of 23 pounds). His A1c dropped to 6.7 and he has signed on for the advanced PNP.

Francine, age 51

Francine is a 51-year-old female who presented with symptoms of insulin resistance and polycystic ovarian syndrome. A realtor and certified drug counselor, Francine is married and the mother of two children. She is 5'3" tall and weighed 230 pounds. Although she had weighed 245 at one point, she was determined to exercise and change her eating habits. She had been on every diet plan out there, never losing more than 30 pounds and always gaining it back (and then some!).

She described herself as a "Pizza Queen and Diet Pepsi Junkie." Francine had bilateral shoulder surgeries four years ago and has ongoing back issues with numbness in her left leg. Her goal is to lose weight, reduce her medication (eventually getting off all prescription medications), and participate in a triathlon. Her periods are irregular. She hasn't had one in over a year and attributes it to steroid use for her back injury. She sees a naprapath regularly.

Francine is on steroids, Hyzaar 225 mg for high blood pressure, and Viactiv for calcium. She also takes a multivitamin, vitamin E, and cinnamon. Her blood pressure is 160/98. She experienced gestational diabetes with her first pregnancy. She exercises regularly to increase her stamina for the triathlon. Her blood work revealed total cholesterol—192 (normal: 5–199); triglycerides—190 (normal: 10–149). Her physician states that triglycerides done in his office were 486; HDL—45 (normal: 40–135); LDL—109 (normal: 0–99).

In ten weeks, Francine weighed in at 193—a loss of 33 pounds. Her blood pressure was 117/78 and her Hyzaar was reduced to 20 mg from 225 mg. Francine's menstrual cycle returned—she has periods once again. At 12 weeks, her blood work improved: total cholesterol—161; triglycerides 172; HDL 35; and LDL—92. Francine has just celebrated her one-year anniversary on the PNP weighing in at 157. She wants to lose 25 more pounds and is successfully on the road to that goal. She is off all medication and no longer buys her clothing in the "plus size" department.

Nancy, age 18

Nancy is an 18-year-old female suffering from poly-cystic ovarian syndrome and pre-diabetes. Her periods were irregular and she had regular outbreaks of acne. She had the typical "pin cushion" look to her face, arms, legs of pancreatic abusers—she was puffy and bloated. Nancy's morning glucose readings ranged from 100 to 140. Many meals that she believed were healthy (sandwiches from a popular sandwich chain) actually raised her blood glucose. For example, after eating turkey on whole wheat with mayo, lettuce, and cucumbers and a glass of water, her blood glucose was 171.

Nancy is 5'1" tall and weighed 141 pounds at her first visit with me. By testing her blood 90 minutes after every meal, she began to understand what foods her pancreas could handle and what foods it could not handle. After six weeks, her skin cleared up and she now weighs 120 pounds. She has more weight to lose. Her goal is to weigh between 110 and 114 pounds.

At the age of 18, she has a road map for the rest of her life. The knowledge Nancy has about foods and healthy eating will continue to enhance and sustain good health.

CHAPTER THIRTEEN

Sample Meal Choices and Recipes

> "There is no food or drink worth poor health."
> — *Candice Rosen*

I LOVE THE **KISS** CONCEPT: "Keep It Simple Stupid." Therefore, I make the food choice options for the PNP program simple. Try to adhere to these types of meals for the first 12 weeks. The following breakfast, lunch, dinner, and snack examples are what I would typically eat.

Each day for the next 12 weeks, mix and match.

Many people believe that if you are a vegan or a vegetarian, you automatically eat healthy. That is not necessarily true. There are many overweight vegetarians and vegans.

Remember, YOUR BODY, YOUR PANCREAS WILL TELL YOU WHAT YOU CAN AND CANNOT EAT! With your blood glucose results in hand (glucose between 70 and 100), you will understand what food is "safe" for you to eat and what food is "unsafe" for you to eat.

The Pancreatic Nutritional Program (PNP)™ is the measurable approach to improved health and weight loss.*

What to Choose at Meals

Breakfast

1. A bowl of fruit (Either cut it up yourself the night before or buy fruit cut up in the produce department of your neighborhood store.)
2. Beverage: decaf coffee, tea, hot water
3. Old-fashioned oatmeal with cinnamon sprinkled on top and unsweetened almond milk
4. One banana
5. One apple
6. Egg-white omelet
7. Scrambled eggs with green pepper, onions, mushrooms
8. Scrambled tofu with any kind of veggies
9. Grape-nuts or grape-nut flakes with unsweetened almond milk

---

*Note: Once the pancreas is in idle mode and you have lost weight and maintained a healthy weight you might be able to add certain items to your diet (example: one slice of rye or whole grain bread with a protein (such as salmon, turkey, tuna, egg or grilled veggies).

10. Boiled egg with veggies
11. Tofu breakfast sausage with scrambled egg whites
12. Salad (easy to just buy the pre-washed, packaged salad—provides 2–3 servings) with ½ avocado. Who says you can't have a salad for breakfast?
13. ½ hemp bagel with non-dairy "cream cheese"
14. A smoothie (Candice's smoothie recipe. The key: include a scoop of "Vega" protein powder). You may have to experiment with various smoothies. This is the rare occasion when you can combine fruit with greens and protein.
15. Zucchini frittata
16. Uncle Sam cereal with unsweetened almond milk
17. Candice's Super Smoothie

Lunch

1. Omelet and salad (veggies, no cheese)
2. Soup (no milk or cream based; no pasta)—may purchase pre-made soups at a local health conscious restaurant, serve with coleslaw (get a bag of pre-chopped coleslaw and add onion powder, garlic powder, sea salt and pepper, sprinkle red wine vinegar or apple cider vinegar and olive oil on top).
3. Lettuce wraps: head of lettuce (gently peel away so the leaves stay intact, rinse and drain). Stir fry onion, peppers, mushrooms, pea pods in a small amount (1 teaspoon) of sesame oil. May also add a seasoning dose of tamari. Then add leftover chicken,

tempeh, or tofu to the mixture and then just place a generous spoonful on the leaf and roll up.

4. Wedge. Cut a generous wedge from a head of lettuce. Rinse it, place it on a plate with tomatoes, cucumbers, and half a can of black beans (rinsed and drained). Oil and vinegar or Brianna's Real French Vinaigrette Dressing.

5. Fajitas without the tortilla, or if you must—ask for lettuce or romaine as a substitute for the tortilla.

6. Hummus with veggies and a Jerusalem salad

7. ½ bag of broccoli slaw and ½ can black beans, add dressing

8. Vegetarian chili

9. Salmon burger grilled with Dijon mustard, with steamed asparagus. After weight and blood work stabilize, you may use one slice of bread (rye or multi-grain).

10. Bean burger with side salad and 2–3 avocado slices

11. Black bean soup with a side salad

12. Steamed, grilled or boiled shrimp served with veggies or a salad

Snacks

1. Celery with almond butter
2. Unsalted tortilla chips with guacamole
3. 10–12 almonds or walnuts (unsalted)
4. Low salt tomato or V-8 juice with celery
5. Apple
6. Banana

7. Pear
8. Bean and avocado salad
9. ½ tart apple with 1 tablespoon of crunchy unsweetened almond butter
10. Candice's Super Smoothie
11. 4–6 shrimp dipped in Dijon mustard
12. Cucumber slices topped with hummus
13. 2–3 asparagus spears wrapped in 1–2 slices of lox

Dinner

1. Tofu and veggies
2. Candice's quick marinara with pasta and arugula salad
3. Pasta with cabbage
4. White bean soup and salad
5. Baked stuffed peppers
6. Salmon (any fish grilled), salad, and steamed asparagus or broccoli
7. Bean and avocado salad
8. Mushroom Bolognese with pasta and a salad
9. Quinoa and veggies
10. Veggie burgers or salmon burgers with sautéed sauerkraut
11. Broccoli slaw with beans and avocado dressing
12. Roasted chicken, veggies, and salad
13. Stew—vegetarian, fish, or chicken
14. Baked sweet potato with a side salad and your favorite vegetable (steamed)

Starter PNP Recipes

Arugula Salad

Arugula (amount depends on how many servings are required)

Sea salt (pinch)
1 lemon
2–3 tablespoons of olive oil

Rinse and drain arugula and place in large bowl.

Sprinkle with pinch of sea salt. Squeeze fresh lemon over the arugula.
Drizzle 2–3 tablespoons of olive oil over arugula.
Adjust lemon, salt and olive oil to taste.

Baked Stuffed Bell Peppers

2 cups cooked grain (brown rice, quinoa, millet, barley). Kasha could be used; however, my family did not like it in this recipe.

1 zucchini chopped

1 onion, finely chopped

2 cloves garlic, finely minced

4 celery stalks, finely chopped

4–6 large bell peppers

½ cup parsley, chopped

1 can organic tomato sauce

1 can diced organic tomatoes

2 teaspoons olive oil or ghee

Salt and pepper to taste

Preheat oven to 350 degrees.

Sauté onion and garlic in oil about 1 min.

Add celery and zucchini, sauté for 3 min.

Mix with remaining ingredients, except peppers and diced tomatoes.

Cut off tops of peppers and gently scoop out insides.

Steam peppers until slightly tender (sometimes I omit this part due to time constraints).

Fill each pepper with stuffing and top with a spoonful of diced tomatoes.

Place in casserole dish with ⅛ inch water, bake for 30 min. (if you didn't steam, then bake for 5 min. more—check for pepper softness).

I cover the peppers with aluminum foil for the first 20–25 minutes and then uncover for the remainder.

Bean and Avocado Salad

⅓ can organic corn (may have to omit; corn may increase your glucose)

1 can organic black beans

1 can organic kidney beans

1 can organic chick peas

2–3 avocados chopped (make sure they are firm, not mushy)

Small bunch of cilantro chopped

2 green onions or ½ leek chopped fine

3–4 tomatoes chopped (make sure they are firm, not mushy)

3 limes

Pinch of sea salt

1–2 tablespoons of olive oil

Rinse and drain all canned items.

In a large bowl, combine all ingredients, sprinkle with sea salt to taste (try to reduce the amount of sodium you use), squeeze the juice from 3 limes on top, add 1–2 tablespoons of olive oil (may need to use a bit more). Toss and serve.

Bean Burger

½ medium onion, chopped

½ teaspoon of cumin

1 clove garlic, chopped fine

2 15-oz. cans of organic black beans, rinsed, drained and partially mashed

2 tablespoons cilantro, chopped

2 teaspoons fresh parsley, chopped

1 teaspoon crushed red pepper

¼ cup oatmeal uncooked

½ cup whole grain bread crumbs

Sea salt and pepper to taste

1–2 tablespoons of olive oil

Pre-heat pan to medium heat. Add one tablespoon of olive oil.

Lightly brown onion and garlic. Take pan off of stove. In a large bowl, combine onions, garlic, beans, and the remaining ingredients. Season with salt and pepper. Mix well.

If it is too wet, add more oatmeal.

If it is too dry, add water one teaspoon at a time.

Divide mixture into 4 equal patties. Place a small amount of olive oil in the pan and cook, browning patties about 6 minutes on each side.

May make ahead and freeze.

You have to use the oatmeal and breadcrumbs with this recipe, otherwise the burger will be mushy. These "carbs" are used in small amounts and only to bind the ingredients for cooking.

Braised Sauerkraut

1–2 jars of Bubbies' sauerkraut rinsed and drained (I double the recipe for leftovers.)

1 medium onion or one large leek (white part)

1 tablespoon chopped garlic

1 teaspoon ghee

Drain and rinse sauerkraut.

Heat large saucepan, melt ghee and add onions or leeks and garlic—lightly brown.

Add sauerkraut, let the sauerkraut brown a bit, scraping brown bits from the bottom of the pan. Heat thoroughly and enjoy.

I make this as a side dish; however, if I want a main dish, I will cut up 1 sweet potato into bite-sized pieces and sauté it along with the onions, etc. After adding the sauerkraut, cover the pan and allow the dish to steam for 5–10 min. until the sweet potatoes are soft, but not mushy.

Broccoli Slaw with Beans and Avocado Dressing

Serves 2–4 (depending on whether it is a main or side dish)

1 bag of broccoli slaw (rinsed and drained)
1 can organic beans (navy, kidney, black, your choice) rinsed and drained

In a large bowl, combine the broccoli slaw and the beans.

Avocado Dressing

¼ cup of fresh lime juice   2 scallions chopped
1 avocado peeled and cut up   ⅓ cup cilantro (chopped)
1 teaspoon of garlic (chopped)   ½ cup olive oil or sunflower oil

In a small bowl, place all ingredients except oil in a blender and puree.
Gradually pour in oil. Blend slowly and season with sea salt.

Candice's Marinara Sauce

1 large can of organic tomato sauce with tomato bits

1 large can of organic tomato sauce

1 large onion

2 tablespoons of chopped garlic

One small bunch of fresh basil chopped

1 tablespoon of anchovy paste

3 tablespoons of olive oil

In large saucepan, heat olive oil. Add onions and garlic and sauté until onions are soft and garlic is slightly brown.

Add the cans of tomatoes.

Add anchovy paste and chopped basil. Make sure the paste is thoroughly blended.

Bring to a boil, then reduce heat and simmer for 20 minutes.

Could also cut up a medium size eggplant and sauté it with onions and garlic (sauté eggplant until it is brown).

Cook pasta according to directions.

Serve pasta marinara with a salad.

Jerusalem Salad

2 servings

1 large cucumber, peeled and diced (about 1½–2 cups)

3 firm plum tomatoes, seeded and diced (about 2 cups)

1 handful parsley, roughly chopped

3 tbsp. tahini (sauce)

Fresh black pepper

½ of a lemon

Pinch of kosher salt

Toss cucumbers, tomatoes, and parsley in a bowl. Add tahini and toss to coat—salad should not be soupy. Grind fresh pepper over the top. Season with an extra dash of salt or a squeeze of lemon if desired. Serve as a side for falafel, or as a refreshing summer side salad. I like to add chopped romaine lettuce to it.

Lemon Tahini Dressing

(Makes ⅔ cup—only about 2 tablespoons is needed for the salad)

Zest of 1 lemon

Juice of 2 lemons (about 4 tablespoons)

2 tablespoons white wine vinegar

¼ cup olive oil

⅓ cup tahini

Salt and pepper to taste

Whisk together all ingredients.

What isn't used can be stored in the refrigerator in a sealed container for up to two weeks.

Baked Falafel
Makes about 18–22 balls

2 15-ounce cans garbanzo beans

1 small onion, finely chopped

2–3 garlic cloves, finely chopped

3 tablespoons fresh parsley, chopped

1 tablespoon fresh cilantro, chopped

1 teaspoon lemon juice

1 teaspoon olive oil

1 teaspoon coriander

1½ teaspoons cumin

½ teaspoon dried red pepper flakes

2 tablespoons whole wheat flour

1 teaspoon baking powder

Kosher or sea salt and pepper to taste

Preheat oven to 375 degrees.

Drain and rinse the garbanzo beans. In a large bowl, mash beans. Combine the rest of the ingredients, adding to the beans, and mix well.

Form into small balls, about the size of golf balls and slightly flatten.

Place onto an oiled baking pan.

Bake for 15 minutes on each side, until nicely browned.

Serve with hummus, tahini sauce, tomatoes, lettuce and/or cucumber or Jerusalem Salad.

Lentil Edamame Salad

1 pkg. of cooked lentils or one can of organic lentils—rinsed and drained (You could cook the lentils yourself.)

1 pkg. ready to eat edamame

¼–⅓ cup of pine nuts

Fresh chopped basil

1–2 tablespoons of olive oil

Mix first four ingredients together and toss with the olive oil.

Mushroom Bolognese

1 pound mushrooms

1 tablespoon olive oil

1 large yellow onion, chopped

2–3 garlic cloves, finely chopped

1 tablespoon tomato paste

1 large can of diced organic tomatoes

3 tablespoons fresh basil, chopped

1 pound whole wheat or brown rice pasta

Salt and pepper to taste

Veggie parmesan cheese (optional)

Slice mushrooms or purchase pre-cut mushrooms. Heat oil in large saucepan. Add onion and garlic—cook for 2–3 minutes. Add mushrooms and cook over high heat for 3–4 minutes stirring occasionally. You will see a lot of liquid. If it appears to be excessive, drain some of the liquid, but not all of it.

Add tomato paste, chopped tomatoes and 1 tablespoon of basil.

Lower heat, cover and cook for 5 minutes.

Cook pasta according to package directions and drain.

Season sauce with salt and pepper. Toss with pasta, sprinkle with remaining basil and serve. Pass around the veggie parmesan. Add an arugula salad dressed with sea salt, lemon and olive oil.

Our Favorite Salad

Whatever you have on hand: head lettuce, romaine, mixed greens

1–2 tomatoes

½ cucumber

½ small red onion

2–3 tablespoons of olive oil

Sea salt to taste

Pepper to taste

Onion powder to taste

Garlic powder to taste

Combine first four ingredients in a large bowl. Sprinkle with onion powder, garlic powder, sea salt, oregano.

Pour ¼ cup of red wine vinegar, white wine vinegar, or apple cider vinegar over salad. Add 3 tablespoons of olive oil. Toss and taste—you may have to add a bit more vinegar or a bit more olive oil.

Pasta with Cabbage and Brussels Sprouts

6 tablespoons of olive oil

1 large onion chopped or 2 leeks chopped (omit green part)

2 cloves garlic finely chopped

1 medium sized cabbage, shredded or chopped

12–14 Brussels sprouts, trimmed and halved

2 tablespoons fresh dill, chopped

1½–2 cups vegetable stock (not broth)

16 oz. whole-wheat pasta or brown rice pasta

Salt and pepper to taste

Heat oil in saucepan, sauté onions and garlic over low heat until onions are soft and garlic begins to brown.

Add the cabbage and Brussels sprouts—cook for 4–5 minutes. Stir in dill. Pour in stock. Cover and simmer for 10 minutes (cabbage and Brussels sprouts should be tender crisp). Salt and pepper to taste.

Boil water while cooking the cabbage. When water is at a full boil, add pasta (cook according to package directions).

Drain pasta, mix with cabbage mixture.

Pea Shoot Wrap

Whole-wheat flax tortillas

Edamame hummus

Organic pea shoots

Jar of roasted peppers

1 tomato chopped

½ cup of chopped cucumber

½ cup romaine lettuce, chopped

Spread some hummus on your tortilla, add the veggies. Roll, slice and eat. (Although this recipe combines the carbs/tortilla with the hummus, it works for most clients.)

Salmon

1–2 tbsp. olive oil

2–4 green onions, whole or 1
  leek sliced

Salmon fillets (one per person)

Salt and pepper to taste

Fresh or dried dill

1 lemon wedge

Pour oil into large grilling pan over medium heat. Wash and trim onions and add to pan. Season salmon with sea salt and pepper and add to pan. Grill until crusty and cooked through (about 10 minutes depending on thickness) but not overdone. Check for doneness by inserting small knife in center; flesh will have changed from dark pink to pale pink. Sprinkle with dill, if used. Drizzle with lemon juice and serve.

Could substitute halibut or any favorite fish.

Another preparation:

Purchase parchment paper. Take one sheet for each piece of fish. Brush paper with olive oil, place salmon on paper and top with your favorite veggies. Sprinkle with salt, pepper and fresh dill. Place a slice of lemon on top. Bring edges of paper together, fold over and secure with a paper clip. Place in a 450-degree pre-heated oven for 10 to 15 minutes. Place fish and parchment paper on serving plate, unseal and enjoy.

Simple Chicken

1 organically fed, humanely
  raised chicken

2 tablespoons of olive oil

2–3 lemons

1–2 garlic cloves

Sea salt

2 tablespoons of oregano

Rinse chicken and place in roasting pan. Pre-heat oven to 400 degrees.

Rub chicken with olive oil and fresh-squeezed lemon juice. After you squeeze lemon over the chicken, place the cut-up lemons inside of the chicken with garlic cloves.

Sprinkle chicken with salt and oregano. Marinate for 20–30 minutes.

Place chicken in oven and reduce heat to 350 degrees. Bake covered for 30 minutes and uncovered for 15 minutes.

While chicken is in the oven, steam asparagus or vegetable of choice. Serve with a salad.

Southwest Quinoa

1 cup of quinoa

2 cups of vegetable broth

In a saucepan, bring vegetable broth to a boil and add quinoa. Cook covered, stirring frequently until broth is absorbed and quinoa appears fluffy. It is just like cooking rice.

1 15 oz. can of organic black beans drained and rinsed

½ cup cilantro chopped

1 pint halved grape tomatoes

1 green pepper chopped

⅓–½ cup of avocado dressing (see page 117)

In a large bowl, combine the beans, cilantro, tomatoes, pepper, quinoa, and dressing. Toss thoroughly.

Serve with a salad.

Barley Salad

½ cup raw barley

1 cup of water

1 cup of vegetable broth

Dressing

½ cup of Brianna's Real French Vinaigrette

2 tablespoons Dijon mustard

1 cup halved or quartered mushrooms

1 cup cut green beans, trimmed and halved

1 cup thinly sliced red or yellow bell peppers

½ cup chopped fresh parsley

1 teaspoons butter or ghee

⅔ cup coarsely chopped walnuts

Using a strainer, rinse the barley and drain. In a small heavy skillet on low heat, roast the barley until fragrant and beginning to brown. Place the barley, water, and broth in a small saucepan, cover, and bring to a simmer. Cook on low heat until most of the liquid has been absorbed and the barley is soft, about 40 minutes.

While the barley cooks, whisk together the dressing and Dijon. In a separate bowl, pour half of the dressing over the mushrooms and set aside. Blanch the green beans for 3 to 4 minutes. Drain and set aside to cool. Combine the bell peppers, parsley, and marinated mushrooms.

In a skillet, heat the butter. When it sizzles, sauté the walnuts until they are coated and the butter begins to brown. Remove from the heat.

When the barley is tender, drain it in a colander. Add the drained barley and the remaining dressing to the serving bowl and mix well. Allow the salad to sit for at least 30 minutes before serving. Before serving, toss the green beans and walnuts into the salad.

Tofu and Veggies

1 package firm tofu, cut into cubes.

Lite soy sauce or tamari

1 package of frozen stir-fry vegetables

Marinate tofu for 20 min. with ¼ to ⅓ cup of lite soy sauce or tamari.

Heat a saucepan and brown tofu cubes 4 minutes on each side.

Transfer tofu to a separate plate or bowl.

Cook frozen vegetables, add tofu and serve. May want to add additional tamari sauce (may substitute shrimp or scallops for tofu).

White Bean Soup

1–2 cans of organic cannellini beans (I don't always have the time to deal with dried beans.)

3 bay leaves

5 tablespoons olive oil

1 large leek (white part) finely chopped

1 carrot, finely chopped (may or may not spike your glucose)

2 celery ribs, finely chopped

3 medium tomatoes, peeled and finely chopped or 1 can diced organic tomatoes

2 cloves garlic, finely chopped

2 teaspoons fresh dill

3 cups vegetable or chicken broth

Salt and pepper to taste

Puree about ¾ of the beans in a food processor along with 1 cup of broth.

Heat oil in a large saucepan. Sauté onion until soft. Add the carrot and celery, cook for 5 minutes more until soft, but not mushy.

Stir in tomatoes, garlic and thyme. Cook for 6–8 minutes, stirring often.

Boil the remaining 2 cups of broth—add the bean puree and the rest of the "whole beans." Salt and pepper to taste. Simmer for 10–15 minutes, allowing flavors to blend.

Serve with a salad and side of vegetables (asparagus or zucchini).

Zucchini Frittata

Serves 6

9- or 10-inch pie plate

3 medium zucchini (approximately 1 lb)

1 leek chopped (white part)

1-2 tbsp extra virgin olive oil

6 large eggs, beaten (organic free-range)

½ cup veggie Parmesan cheese

6 fresh basil leaves chopped

Salt and pepper to taste

In an 8-inch ovenproof skillet over medium heat, sauté leek and zucchini in oil for 2-3 minutes. Pour eggs over top; sprinkle with minimal salt and pepper. Cook until almost set, 5-6 minutes. Sprinkle with cheese. Bake at 350 degrees F. for 40-45 minutes or until the cheese is melted or the top begins to brown.

Arugula and Lentil Salad

Arugula (large bag, organic)

8 stalks of asparagus

1 can of lentils, drained

Sea salt

Juice from 1–2 lemons

2–3 tablespoons of olive oil

Veggie Parmesan cheese

Rinse arugula. Rinse and drain lentils. Blanch asparagus and cut into ½-inch pieces.

Combine. Sprinkle small amount of sea salt over salad, add lemon juice, olive oil and toss.

Candice's Super Smoothie

1 scoop of Vega protein powder (scoop is in the container)

½ cup of blueberries

½ banana (I peel, cut bananas in half and freeze—makes it so much easier.)

1 cup of kale (cut up)

1 cup of romaine (cut up)

4–5 ice cubes

1 cup of unsweetened almond milk

The only way I can drink a smoothie is if I put protein powder in it. Otherwise, a smoothie will raise my blood sugar well above 100. Example: smoothie without protein powder: glucose—126; with protein powder: glucose—84.

Resources

Integrative Nutrition by Joshua Rosenthal
The China Study by Dr. T. Colin Campbell
Diet for a Small World by Frances Moore Lappé
Prevent and Reverse Heart Disease by Caldwell B.
    Esselstyn, Jr., M.D.
The Omnivore's Dilemma by Michael Pollan
Take Charge of Your Diabetes by Sarfraz Zaidi, M.D.
Stay Healthy with Nutrition by Elson M. Haas, M.D. with
    Buck Levin, PhD.
The State of Health Atlas by Diarmuid O'Donovan
*The New Glucose Revolution, What Makes My Blood Glucose
    Go Up and Down?* by Dr. Jennie Brand-Miller
Vegetarian Cooking for Everyone by Deborah Madison
Kundalini Yoga DVD by Maya Fiennes

Callanetics 10 Years Younger in 10 Hours by Callan
  Pinckney
Movies: *Food, Inc.* (incredibly informative and thought
  provoking), *Forks over Knives* and *Wall-E*
The Pancreatic Oath Online Nutrition Journal—
  www.ilovemypancreas.com
LOCALI—www.localiyours.com
Pancreatic Nutritional Program (PNP)™—
  www.pnprogram.com

Glossary

Arteriosclerosis—Thickening of the walls of the arterioles with loss of elasticity and contractility.

Atherosclerosis—A form of arteriosclerosis in which there are localized accumulations of lipid-containing material within or beneath the intimal surfaces of blood vessels.

Cholesterol—A sterol (one of a group of substances related to fats and belonging to the lipoids) widely distributed in animal tissues and occurring in the yolk of eggs, various oils, fats, and nerve tissue (brain and spinal cord). It can be synthesized in the liver and is a normal constituent of bile. It is the principal constituent of most gallstones (80%). It is important in metabolism, serving as a precursor of various steroid hormones, e.g. sex hormones, adrenal corticoids, etc. Normal range: 125–200 mg/dL.

Diabetes—A condition in which a person has a high blood sugar (glucose) level, either because the body doesn't produce enough insulin, or because body cells don't properly respond to the insulin that is produced. Insulin is a hormone produced in the pancreas which enables body cells to absorb glucose, to turn it into energy. If the body cells do not absorb the glucose, the glucose will accumulate in the blood (hyperglycemia), leading to vascular, nerve, and other complications.

There are many types of diabetes, the most common of which are:

+ **Type 1 diabetes:** results from the body's failure to produce insulin; presently requires the person to inject insulin.
+ **Type 2 diabetes:** results from insulin resistance, a condition in which cells fail to use insulin properly, sometimes combined with an absolute insulin deficiency.
+ **Gestational diabetes:** is when pregnant women, who have never had diabetes before, have a high blood glucose level during pregnancy. It may precede development of Type 2 diabetes.

FSH (Follicle stimulating hormone)—Secreted by the anterior lobe of the hypothalamus, which in turn stimulates the development of the ovarian follicles.

HDL (High density lipoprotein; "good cholesterol")—About one-fourth to one-third of blood cholesterol is carried by high-density lipoprotein (HDL). HDL cholesterol is known as "good" cholesterol, because high levels of HDL seem to protect against heart attack. Low levels of HDL (less than 40 mg/dL) also increase the risk of heart disease. Medical experts think that HDL tends to carry cholesterol away from the arteries and back to the liver, where it's passed from the body. Some experts believe that HDL removes excess cholesterol from arterial plaque. Normal: > or = 40 mg/dL.

Hyperinsulinism—Excessive amount of insulin in the blood. Excessive sensitivity to an increase in blood sugar level.

Insulin Resistance—Insulin resistance is a condition in which cells, particularly those of muscle, fat, and liver tissue, display "resistance" to insulin by failing to take up and utilize glucose for energy and metabolism (insulin normally promotes take up and utilization of blood glucose from the bloodstream). In its early stages, the condition is asymptomatic, but may develop into Type 2 diabetes. Although there are several established risk factors, the underlying cause is unknown.

It has been estimated that 30 to 33 million Americans are insulin resistant, and the number appears to be increasing.

LDL (Low-density lipoprotein; "bad cholesterol")— When too much LDL (bad) cholesterol circulates in the blood, it can slowly build up in the inner walls of the arteries that feed the heart and brain. Together with other substances, it can form plaque, a thick, hard deposit that can narrow the arteries and make them less flexible. This condition is known as atherosclerosis. If a clot forms and blocks a narrowed artery, heart attack or stroke can result. Normal: < 130 mg/dL.

LH (luteinizing hormone)—induces ovulation and the formation of the corpus luteum (principal part of a small yellow body, which develops within a ruptured ovarian follicle).

It is an endocrine structure secreting progesterone. Also stimulates development of interstitial cells of the testes.

Metabolic Syndrome—Metabolic syndrome is when a person has a group of metabolic risk factors including:

+ Abdominal obesity (excessive fat tissue in and around the abdomen)
+ Blood fat disorders (mainly high triglycerides and low HDL cholesterol that foster plaque buildups in artery walls)

+ Insulin resistance or glucose intolerance (the body can't properly use insulin or blood sugar)
+ Prothrombotic state (e.g., high fibrinogen or plasminogen activator inhibitor [–1] in the blood)
+ Raised blood pressure (130/85 mm Hg or higher)
+ Pro-inflammatory state (e.g., elevated high-sensitivity C-reactive protein in the blood). The underlying causes of metabolic syndrome are overweight/obesity, physical inactivity, and genetic factors. People with metabolic syndrome are at increased risk of coronary heart disease, other diseases related to plaque buildups in artery walls (e.g., stroke and peripheral vascular disease) and Type 2 diabetes.

Omnivore—An omnivorous person or animal. Omnivorous—feeding on every kind of food available; eating both plant and animal food.

Obesity—Abnormal amount of fat on the body. Two classifications:

    Exogenous—caused by excessive food intake.

    Endogenous (coming from within)—caused by some abnormality within the body (endocrine or faulty metabolism). Endocrine causes: hypothyroidism (frequently used as an excuse for weight gain); adrenal hyperfunction; testicular and ovarian hypofunction.

Pancreatic Abuse—When the consumption of food portions and/or poor choices outweighs or exceeds the capability of the pancreas.

Polycystic ovarian syndrome—The principal features are obesity, anovulation (resulting in irregular menstruation), acne, and excessive amounts or effects of androgenic (masculinizing) hormones. The symptoms and severity of the syndrome vary greatly among women. While the causes are unknown, insulin resistance, diabetes, and obesity are all strongly correlated with PCOS.

Pre-diabetes—Pre-diabetes is the state that occurs when a person's blood glucose levels are higher than normal, but not high enough for a diagnosis of diabetes. About 11% of people with pre-diabetes in the Diabetes Prevention Program standard or control group developed Type 2 diabetes each year during the average three years of follow-up. Other studies show that many people with pre-diabetes develop Type 2 diabetes in 10 years.

Triglycerides—Triglyceride is a form of fat made in the body. Elevated triglycerides can be due to overweight/obesity, physical inactivity, cigarette smoking, excess alcohol consumption and a diet very high in carbohydrates (60% of total calories or more). People with high triglycerides often have a high total cholesterol level, including a high LDL (bad) level and a low HDL (good) level. Many people with heart disease and/or diabetes also have high triglyceride levels. Normal: < 150 mg/dL.

Vegetarian—A person who on principle abstains from animal food; especially one who avoids meat, but will consume dairy products and eggs and sometimes also fish. Living wholly or largely on vegetables or plants.

Vegan—A total vegetarian, i.e. one who avoids dairy products and eggs as well as meat and fish.

Annotated Bibliography

1. Haas, Elson M., M.D. *Staying Healthy with Nutrition.* Celestial Arts, 2006, p. 30.
2. Ibid.
3. Ibid.
4. Cancer. Fact Sheet No 297, 2009. World Health Organization. Available at http://www.who.int/media centre/factsheets/fs297/en/print.html. Accessed Feb 8, 2011.
5. Ibid.
6. Diabetes Home. National Diabetes Information Clearinghouse (NDIC), National Institutes of Diabetes and Digestive and Kidney Disease, National Institute of Health. http://diabetes.niddk.nih.gov/about/index/htm.

7. The Voice of Clinical Endocrinology. American Association of Clinical Endocrinologists. http://media.aace.com/article_display.cfm?article_id=4828. Accessed August 2009.

8. The Voice of Clinical Endocrinology. American Association of Clinical Endocrinologists. http://media.aace.com/article_display.cfm?article_id=4828. Accessed August 2009.

9. Center for Disease Control and Prevention. National Center for Health Statistics, http://www.cdc.gov/nchs/fastats/diabetes.htm. Accessed February 2008.

10. Giovannucci, E., D.M. Harlan, M.C. Archer et al. "Diabetes and Cancer: A Consensus Report." *CA Cancer J Clin* 2010; 60(4):207–221.

11. O'Donovan, Diarmuid. *The State of Health Atlas.* University of California Press, 2008, p. 48.

12. Kim, J. W., and C. V. Dang. "Cancer's molecular sweet tooth and the Warburg effect." *Cancer Res.* 66.18 (2006): 8927-30.

13. Center for Disease Control and Prevention. National Center for Health Statistics. http://www.cdc.gov/nchs/fastats/diabetes.htm. Accessed February 2008.

14. Ibid.

15. Khan, M.S., Ph.D., Alam, Safdar, M.S., Mahpara, Ali Khan, M.S., Ph.D., Mohammad Muzaffar, Khattak, M.S., Khan Nawaz, and Anderson, Ph.D., Richard A., "Cinnamon Improves Glucose and Lipids of People with Type 2 Diabetes." *Diabetes Care* 26 (2003): 3215–18.

Additional Sources

American Diabetes Association
The American Heart Association
The Shorter Oxford English Dictionary
Davis, Clayton, Thomas, M.D., *Taber's Cyclopedic Medical Dictionary*, F.A. Davis Company, Philadelphia
http://en.wikipedia.org/wiki/Polycystic_ovary_syndrome-cite_note-3
http://en.wikipedia.org/wiki/Diabetes_mellitus
http://www.worlddiabetesday.org/files/docs/Economic_aspects.pdf

About the Author

Candice Rosen, R.N., B.S., M.S.W., C.H.C.
Founder, Executive Director and Principal PNP™
Health Counselor

As a Registered Nurse with a Master's Degree in Social Work and Certification in Health Counseling from the Institute for Integrative Nutrition, Candice Rosen has spent her life's work focused on improving the wellness of both her clients and her community. Her experiences as a clinical therapist and as a nurse give her a unique perspective when it comes to nutrition counseling. Candice has an innate understanding of the medical and psychological components that must be addressed in order to achieve health goals and targeted weight loss results.

As the founding member of Gilda's Club Chicago and its first executive director and program director, Candice created and coordinated a diverse array of wellness-related programming. Now Chair of Healthcare Initiatives for Chicago's Sister Cities International Program, she works to advocate preventive medicine, increase maternal and infant health care, improve disability access, promote nourishing diets, and bring awareness to the obesity and diabetes epidemics that now affects populations on a global level.

The originator and director of the Pancreatic Nutritional Program™ (PNP™), Candice is also on a mission to educate the general public as to the crucial role the pancreas plays in overall health, wellness and maintaining an optimal weight. She was inspired to write this, her second book, *The Pancreatic Oath* (Spring 2011), based on her experience helping many clients with conditions such as diabetes, cardiovascular disease, obesity, metabolic syndrome, polycystic ovarian syndrome, and kidney disease. She has helped to manage and often reverse their symptoms through her innovative Pancreatic Nutritional Program™. Too often the accepted method of practice is to treat symptoms with prescription drugs, while ignoring underlying causes. The PNP™ and this book focus on the underlying causes, specifically pancreatic abuse, and treat the source of illness rather than the consequences. While Candice stresses that there is no such thing as a "one size fits all" diet, she has developed a program that benefits all who practice it.

EDUCATION

Institute For Integrative Nutrition and the State University of New York (SUNY), New York City, New York—Certified Health Coach

Loyola University, Chicago, Illinois—Master of Social Work

University of St. Francis, Joliet, Illinois—Bachelor of Science

South Chicago Community Hospital School of Nursing, Chicago, Illinois—Registered Nurse

LICENSURE

Licensed Social Worker—State of Illinois

Licensed Registered Nurse—State of Illinois

PROFESSIONAL AND COMMUNITY INVOLVEMENT

Chairman, Healthcare Initiatives, Chicago Sister Cities International Program

Board of Directors, Chicago Sister Cities International Program

Member, Access Living's Major Gifts Campaign Committee

Member, Ambassador Council, Center for Integrative Medicine and Wellness, Northwestern University Medical Center

Board Member, Face the Future Foundation

Member, International Women's Association

Member, American Association of Drugless Practitioners

Member, American Holistic Nurses Association
Member, American Nurses Association
Member, Illinois Nurses Association
Member, National Association of Social Workers
Member, Illinois Society of Clinical Social Work
Member, Illinois Mental Health Association
Member, Association Oncology Social Work
Member, Oncology Nurses Society
Member, Northwestern University Circle Club
Member, Evanston and Glenbrook Hospital Auxiliary
Honoree, Notable Alumni—University of St. Francis 90th
    Anniversary Celebratory Magazine

FAMILY
Candice and her husband, Steven, have four children, a Portuguese water dog, an African Grey Parrot, and a Red-Eared Slider Turtle.

Acknowledgements

The Pancreatic Oath is the result of a mother's quest to help her daughter. Combining information from a constellation of research sources to create a nutrition program (that evolved into a book) was never the intent, but it has been a miraculous process!

I have so many generous people to thank and I am so grateful to the many teachers who have crossed my path.

Thank you to my first guinea pig, my daughter Jennifer. Her symptoms caused frustration and discomfort and the need to find a solution. To my daughter Natalie, who was "strong armed" into following the Pancreatic Nutritional Program (PNP); thank you for now being its biggest cheerleader. To my son, Nicholas, who once had to be forcefully persuaded to at least try *something green* as a pre-teen; you have now become my first source for the latest news on fitness and diet. Your transformation from a fast food junkie kid into a model for healthy living and eating serves as the ultimate inspiration for me.

To Ginna, for seeing the change in me and asking for help. Her metamorphosis opened up the door for Sally and Pamela. Their quest for Self-Health has not only improved their health, but also increased their quality of life. Thank you for being the "poster children" of the PNP and spreading the message. Thank you to Alex, for addressing your health issues early on.

There are many individuals to thank: Linda Beckstrom, Bonnie Sweet, Gail Parke, and Laurie Harris; and many others who have inspired me: Loretta Roberts, Dr. T. Colin Campbell, Joshua Rosenthal, Dr. Carl Esselstyn, Jean Wright, and Maya Fiennes.

I owe immeasurable gratitude to my daughter Melissa. As my first born, she has always been a believer of Mom and my biggest fan. Melissa, along with her husband Greg, paved the way for me and the Rosen family to venture off the "comfort/junk food" road to one filled with nutritious, wholesome food and improved health. Melissa has been my right hand, working alongside me with clients and taking my book and the PNP to the next level.

To Michael Sapko, for editing and assisting in the final draft of *The Pancreatic Oath*. Thank you for "getting me," *The Pancreatic Oath* and the PNP. I look forward to the next project.

To Michele DeFilippo, Ronda Rawlins, Amy Collins, Carrie Simons, Ashley Sandberg, Todd Stephens, Taylor

Erdman, Zareen Jaffery, Derek Nelson, Ted Novak and Jane Moroney, for helping me deliver my message. I am deeply grateful.

Thank you to my father Robert Polovina and my late mother, Nada—wish I knew then what I know now.

And finally, my dear husband, Steven, who was dragged along the PNP path kicking and screaming. His understanding of vegetarianism was "dates wrapped in bacon!" Change is hard. He has come a long way from "medical model" thinking to a more "holistic" approach to healthcare. I am proud of him.

Finally, I would like to thank the human body, in particular the pancreas, for "functioning" under the most difficult circumstances.

Index

CPSIA information can be obtained at www.ICGtesting.com
Printed in the USA
LVOW062117101011

249941LV00002B/8/P